THE
CODE
BREAKER

THE
CODE
BREAKER

UNLOCKING THE MYSTERIES OF HEALTH AND VITALITY
AND ESTABLISHING THE FOUNDATION FOR A DISEASE-FREE LIFE

DR. ANDY BARLOW, D.C.

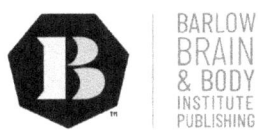

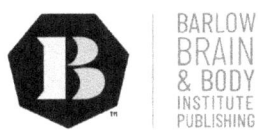

BARLOW
BRAIN
& BODY
INSTITUTE
PUBLISHING

To the love of my life, Faye Barlow.

This book is dedicated to you, my rock, my inspiration, and my unwavering support throughout the past 35 years. From our humble beginnings at Cooper Tire, where we both worked and pursued our education, to my journey at Life University and the Carrick Institute of Functional Neurology, you have been by my side every step of the way.

From the countless 4 am early-morning study sessions to seemingly endless seminars, traveling weekends from one city to the next attending them, as well as teaching for the Barlow Brain and Body Institute, it has all been possible because of your unwavering love and belief in me. Your encouragement and understanding have propelled me forward, pushing me to achieve more than I ever thought possible.

You are not only my partner in life but also my biggest cheerleader and confidante. Your love has fueled my passion, and I owe every success I have achieved to you. Without you, there would be no Dr. Andy Barlow.

To the world, I want to declare that beside every great man is an even greater woman. Your unwavering support and love have been the foundation upon which I have built my dreams. Your presence in my life has made me a better person, a better doctor, and a better human being.

Faye, my love, I dedicate this book to you with all my heart. May its words inspire others as you have inspired me. Thank you for being the love of my life, my wife, and my best friend.

Forever yours,
Andy

"That is why I use these parables, For they look, but they don't really see. They hear, but they don't really listen or understand. This fulfills the prophecy of Isaiah that says, 'When you hear what I say, you will not understand. When you see what I do, you will not comprehend. For the hearts of these people are hardened, and their ears cannot hear, and they have closed their eyes-so their eyes cannot see, and their ears cannot hear, and their hearts cannot understand, and they cannot turn to me and let me heal them.'"

MATTHEW 13:13-15

TABLE OF CONTENTS

PART THREE:
UNDERSTANDING YOUR NEXT STEPS

FOREWORD

*"Then you shall know the truth, and
the truth shall set you free."*

JOHN 8:32

I am writing this foreword because I have spent more than 50 years of my life identifying the root causes of many immune disorders, which is in line with the functional medicine and functional neurology that are at the core of this book. I have been part of functional medicine since its inception in 1992. My own particular field of interest is immunology, specializing in systems immunology and autoimmunity.

With the above in mind, I have to say that there is so much in Dr. Barlow's book that resonates with me, because I have thought those same thoughts, I believe those same beliefs, and I hold to those same truths. In almost every chapter I have found something that could have come from my own heart, and I am delighted that he manages to say it with such clarity and wit.

This book was written for and, I hope, will be read and used by medical doctors, chiropractors, naturopaths, nurse practitioners, other members of the medical field, and patients. To all of them and their families I say, "Read Dr. Andy Barlow's book." I would go further, and advise medical practitioners to buy extra copies of this book and give them to their patients. Because who doesn't want a disease-free life?

That's what Dr. Barlow offers in the very subtitle of his book. You may ask, why is the main title "The Code Breaker?" I would hate to spoil the book for anyone, so I'll try to be as general as I can, but there is just so much good material in this book that I just can't help but mention a few things. "The Code Breaker" is about breaking the code of complex diseases that medical practitioners find hard to understand or decipher its source or cause. With the diseases that plague humanity today, a patient may go from doctor to doctor, and each doctor may order a different barrage of tests leading to five or ten different diagnoses, which result in the prescription of five or ten different sets of prescriptions. In the end all the tests are just one big fishing expedition with a big stack of results as the only catch, and, as Dr. Barlow has also said, perhaps the patient is told it's all in their head, or they just have to treat the symptoms, not the actual disease, or they just have to live with it.

For me, a Code Breaker is someone who can decode all the clutter that is obfuscating the management of a patient's disease. The Code Breaker can see clues and hints in a patient's history and symptoms and understand the need for a reliable and accurate lab with the highest standards. The Code Breaker must know which tests to order, because in many cases ordering a single test isn't enough, and sometimes you have to order a comprehensive repertoire of tests. And, finally, the Code Breaker must know how to interpret the results of those tests and break the code of the patient's disease.

Dr. Andy Barlow is the quintessential Code Breaker. He understands his material so well that he can break it down so that even laymen can benefit from reading his book. I recommend everyone not to skip the introduction as some readers do, because it is educational, scientific, spiritual and inspiring. Yes, all that in just the introduction. He also lists in this section the top six causes of death due to chronic illness in the United States: heart disease, cancer, chronic lower respiratory disease, stroke, Alzheimer's disease, and diabetes. These particularly struck me as an immunologist, because all these diseases are connected to the immune and nervous system. They have been the top killers for 20 years, and the medical profession needs to wake up and do something about it!

So why did Dr. Barlow write this book? Who is it for?

In the larger sense, it's for all of us, but it is especially for those who have seen doctor after doctor, taken test after test, undergone treatment after treatment, and still find themselves suffering, and think they have no options and nowhere to turn.

Turn to Dr. Barlow and this book.

Dr. Barlow says the goal of his book is to

1. Enhance your cognitive function while improving your short and long-term memory, organization, and multitasking skills.
2. Optimize your focus, attention, and concentration.
3. Sharpen your memory.
4. Improve your mobility (moving your body) and gut motility (moving food products through your gastrointestinal tract with proper absorption and elimination).

I completely agree with and endorse these goals. As an immunologist, I know that they will contribute towards a properly functioning and healthy immune system.

In Chapter One of this book, Dr. Barlow deals with the brain and its central role in our health and our very existence. He calls the frontal lobe of the brain the gateway to cognition. Indeed, humankind seems to instinctively understand the importance of that part of the brain. Jews bind teffilin boxes or phylacteries on their foreheads for their morning prayers. Muslims bow and touch their foreheads to the turbah (Arabic) or mohr (Farsi) stone in their prayers. Catholics make the sign of the Cross with ashes on their foreheads on Ash Wednesday.

Dr. Barlow talks in this chapter about the connection between the brain and the gut, calling the gut the second brain. He discussed the impact of this brain-gut connection on various aspects of our overall health. I have written about the same thing in my own publications, additionally linking the brain and the gut with the immune system in what I call the gut-brain-immune axis. My own research has shown that someone with a leaky gut is 70% likely to have a leaky brain as well. This chapter is important as we should all realize that what we eat doesn't just affect our stomachs, but can have grave effects on our brains and immune systems as well.

This chapter is where I encountered the first of Dr. Barlow's case reports. And this is where I must say how delighted I am in the way he presents all the case reports or patient's success stories in this book. They are honestly a joy to read. They are brief, clear, informative, highly educational, and somehow, there is this very human element that comes across with each one that makes you care about the patients and see them as more than just a medical statistic.

Another thing I love is the pithy little sayings at the beginning of each chapter, or even those spread liberally throughout the book. Like, "Do one thing every day that scares you." This is the saying that starts Chapter Two, "The Power of a Code," where you learn exactly why this book is about codes and Code Breakers.

Dr. Barlow says that there are specific codes that can unlock the mysteries of chronic health problems, and his book was written to reveal these codes and help us unlock them to give us the healthy life we deserve. Specifically, he says there are seven "codes" or metabolic factors that contribute to the development and progression of complex chronic illnesses.

One thing he says in his book that I really appreciate is that an important part of breaking or interpreting these codes is bloodwork, specific metabolic testing, because, as another of the pithy sayings goes, "If we don't test, it's only a guess." I really loved this one, because my whole adult life and career has basically been about the importance of accurate, reliable testing. In a later chapter, Dr. Barlow says, "We go into these tests with zero bias or preconceived ideas. We do the lab work and let the results tell the story. These tests quantify and objectify reality."

Another thing I really loved was the lasagna analogy. You should read the whole thing to really appreciate it, but it's Dr. Barlow's very apt explanation for why there's no one single test or one single treatment for complex chronic diseases, because they are multivariate or multifactorial, and thus require a multimodal approach with both neurological and metabolic interventions. This is something I heartily endorse because I wrote about this same subject many years ago.

There is also the part where Dr. Barlow talks about "holism" versus "reductionism. If you don't like puns, please forgive me, but I just have to say that it should be a real "eye-opener" for many when Dr. Barlow talks about the two kinds of "lenses" that health practitioners wear when looking at a patient's problems. This part is exciting for me, because this part is directly related to the new fields of systems biology and systems immunology that are making waves in the medical and scientific circles.

There is so much I love about this book. I love how he explains molecular mimicry by having us think of him, whose name is ANDY, being confused with another person named ANDI. And I've already mentioned how I really liked how he presented his case reports or "patient success stories" as he called them, but it really struck me when he disclosed how it was his wife Faye's own struggle with autoimmune disease that led him to study metabolic testing and functional medicine in the first place. This really struck a chord with me, because it was my own mother's suffering from rheumatoid arthritis that inspired me to take the path of immunology. But I had to laugh at the "hockey puck" biscuits, and I'm sure you will too when you get to it.

I am seriously in danger of letting this foreword turn into a review or summary article, so let me wrap this up by saying that I love everything about this book, the writing style, the case reports, the wise and witty sayings, the analogies, but, most of all, the vitally important information and messages that it contains. This part is serious, and we all need to read this book for the sake of our own health.

I wish that Dr. Barlow lived in Los Angeles, because I would have no hesitation in making him my family doctor.

Aristo Vojdani, PhD, MSc, CLS
CEO, Immunosciences Lab., Inc.
Chief Scientific Advisor, Cyrex Labs, LLC

REFERENCES:

1. Vojdani A, editor. Neuroimmunity and the Brain-Gut Connection. *Functional Neurology* series, Nova Science Publishers Inc., New York, 2015.

2. Vojdani A, Tarash I. Cross-reaction between gliadin and different food and tissue antigens. *Food and Nutrition Sciences*, 44:20-32, 2013.

3. Perlmutter D, Vojdani A. Association between headache and sensitivities to gluten and dairy. *Integrative Medicine*, 12(2):39-44, 2013.

4. Vojdani A. Brain-reactive antibodies in traumatic brain injury. *Functional Neurology, Rehabilitation, and Ergonomics*, 3(2-3):173-181, 2013.

5. Vojdani A, Kharrazian D, Mukherjee PS. The prevalence of antibodies against wheat and milk proteins in blood donors and their contribution to neuroautoimmune reactivities. *Nutrients*, 6:15-36, 2014, doi:10.3390/nu6010015, PMID: 24451306

6. Vojdani A. A potential link between environmental triggers and autoimmunity. *Autoimmune Diseases*, Volume 2014, Article ID 437231, 18 pages. http://dx.doi.org/10.1155/2014/437231, 2014, PMID: 24688790

7. Burazor I, Vojdani A. Chronic exposure to oral pathogens and autoimmune reactivity in acute coronary thrombosis. *Autoimmune Diseases*, Volume 2014, Article ID 613157, 8 pages. http://dx.doi.org/10.1155/2014/613157, 2014, PMID: 24839554

8. Vojdani A. Food immune reactivity and neuroautoimmunity. *Funct Neurol Rehabil Ergon*, 4(2-3):175-195, 2014.

9. Calderón-Garcidueñas L., Vojdani A., Blaurock-Busch E., Busch Y., Friedle A., Franco-Lira M., Sarathi-Mukherjee P., Park S.-B., Torres-Jardón R., D'Angiulli A. Air pollution and children: Neural and tight junction antibodies and combustion metals, the role of barrier breakdown, and brain immunity in neurodegeneration. *Journal of Alzheimer's Disease*, 43(3):1039-1058, 2015. doi: 10.3233/JAD-141365, PMID: 25147109

10. Calderón-Garcidueñas L, Gónzalez-Maciel A, Vojdani A, Franco-Lira M, Reynoso-Robles R, Montesinos-Correa H, Pérez-Guillé B, Mukherjee PS, Torres-Jardón R, Calderón-Garcidueñas A and Perry G. The intestinal barrier in air pollution-associated neural involvement in Mexico City residents: mind the gut, the evolution of a changing paradigm relevant to Parkinson disease risk. *J Alzheimers Dis Parkinsonism*, 5(1), 2015, http://dx.doi.org/10.4172/2161-0460.1000179.

11. Vojdani A, Kharrazian D, Mukherjee PS. Elevated levels of antibodies against xenobiotics in a subgroup of healthy subjects. *Journal of Applied Toxicology*, 35(4): 383-397, 2015. doi: 10.1002/jat.3031, PMID: 25042713

12. Vojdani A, Mukherjee PS, Berookhim J, Kharrazian D. Detection of antibodies against human and plant aquaporins in patients with multiple sclerosis. *Autoimmune Diseases*, Volume 2015, Article ID 905208, 10 pages, http://dx.doi.org/10.1155/2015/905208, 2015, PMID: 26290755

13. Vojdani A, Vojdani E. Gluten and non-gluten proteins of wheat as target antigens in autism, Crohn's and celiac disease. *J Cereal Science*, 75: 252-260, 2017.

14. Vojdani A, Vojdani E, Kharrazian D. Fluctuation of zonulin levels in blood versus stability of antibodies. *World J*

Gastroenterol, 23(31): 5669-5679, 2017, doi: 10.3748/wjg. v23.i31.5669, PMID: 28883692

15. Vojdani A, Vojdani E, Saidara E, Kharrazian D (2018) Reaction of amyloid-β peptide antibody with different infectious agents involved in Alzheimer's disease. *J Alzheimers Dis,* 63(2018): 847-860. doi:10.3233/JAD-170961, PMID: 29689721

16. Vojdani A, Vojdani E (2018) Amyloid-β 1-42 cross-reactive antibody prevalent in human sera may contribute to intraneuronal deposition of AβP-42. *Int J Alzheimers Dis* Volume 2018, Article ID 1672568, 12 pages doi:10.1155/2018/1672568, PMID: 30034864

17. Vojdani A, Vojdani E (2018) Immunoreactivity of Anti-AβP-42 specific antibody with toxic chemicals and food antigens. *J Alzheimers Dis Parkinsonism* 8(3):441 doi:10.4172/2161-0460.1000441

18. Vojdani A, Turnpaugh C, Vojdani E (2018) Immune reactivity against a variety of mammalian and plant-based milk substitutes. *J Dairy Research* 85(3): 358-365. doi. org/10.1017/S0022029918000523, PMID: 30156521

19. Vojdani A (2019) Is there a possible correlation between antibodies against lipopolysaccharides, intestinal and blood brain barrier proteins in IBD subjects? *Autoimmun Rev* 18(6):639-641. doi: 10.1016/j.autrev.2019.01.001, PMID: 30959215

20. Kharrazian D, Herbert M, Vojdani A (2019) The associations between immunological reactivity to the haptenation of unconjugated bisphenol A to albumin and protein disulfide isomerase with alpha-synuclein antibodies. *Toxics* 7(2):26 doi: 10.3390/toxics7020026, PMID: 31064082

21. Maes M, Sirivichayakul S, Kanchanatawan B, Vojdani A (2019) Breakdown of the paracellular tight and adherens junctions in the gut and blood brain barrier and damage to the vascular barrier in patients with deficit schizophrenia. *Neurotox Res*, 36(2):306-322. doi:10.1007/s12640-019-00054-6, PMID: 31077000

22. Vojdani A. Reaction of food-specific antibodies with different tissue antigens. *Int J Food Sci Tech*, 55(4):1800-1815, 2020. doi.org/10.1111/ijfs.14467

23. Vojdani A, Gushgari LR, Vojdani E. Interaction between food antigens and the immune system: Association with autoimmune disorders. *Autoimmun Rev*, 19(3):102459, 2020. doi.org/10.1016/j.autrev.2020.102459, PMID: 31917265

24. Vojdani A, Afar D, Vojdani E. Reaction of lectin-specific antibody with human tissue: Possible contributions to autoimmunity. *J Immunol Res*, 2020, vol. 2020, Article ID 1438957, doi: 10.1155/2020/1438957, PMID: 32104714

25. Vojdani A, Vojdani E, Herbert M, Kharrazian D (2020) Correlation between antibodies to bacterial lipopolysaccharides and barrier proteins in sera positive for ASCA and ANCA. *Int J Mol Sci*, 21(4), 1381, doi: 10.3390/ijms21041381, PMID: 32085663

26. Kharrazian D, Herbert M, Vojdani A (2020) Cross-reactivity between chemical antibodies formed to serum proteins and thyroid axis target sites. *Int J Mol Sci*, 21(19), 7324, doi: 10.3390/ijms21197324.

27. Vojdani A, Monro J, Lanzisera F, Sadeghi H. Serological cross-reactivity between viruses and their contribution to autoimmunity. *Autoimmun Rev*, 20:102840, 2021.

28. Vojdani A. Elevated IgG antibody to aluminum bound to human serum albumin in patients with Crohn's, Celiac and

Alzheimer's disease. *Toxics*, 9(9):212, 2021 doi: 10.3390/ toxics9090212.

29. Vojdani A, Vojdani E. The role of exposomes in the pathophysiology of autoimmune diseases I: Toxic chemicals and food. *Pathophysiology*, 28:513-543, 2021.

30. Vojdani A, Vojdani E, Rosenberg AZ, Shoenfeld Y. The role of exposomes in the pathophysiology of autoimmune diseases II: Pathogens. *Pathophysiology*, 29(2):243-280, 2022.

31. Maes M, Thisayakorn P, Thipakorn Y, Tantavisut S, Sirivichayakul S, Vojdani A. Reactivity to neural tissue epitopes, aquaporin 4 and heat shock protein 60 is associated with activated immune-inflammatory pathways and the onset of delirium following hip fracture surgery. *Eur Geriatric Med* (EGEM), 2022, Dec 15. doi: 10.1007/ s41999-022-00729-y.

32. Lavi Y, Vojdani A, Halpert G, Sharif K, Ostrinski Y, Zyskind I, Lattin MT, Zimmerman J, Silverberg JI, Rosenberg AZ, Shoenfeld Y, Amital H. Dysregulated levels of circulating autoantibodies against neuronal and nervous system autoantigens in COVID-19 patients. *Diagnostics*, 2023, 13(4):687, doi: 10.3390/diagnostics13040687.

33. Lerner A, Benzvi C, Vojdani A. SARS-CoV-2 gut-targeted epitopes: Sequence similarity and cross-reactivity join together for molecular mimicry. *Biomedicines*, 2023, 11(7):1937, doi: 10.3390/biomedicines11071937.

34. Lerner A, Benzvi C, Vojdani A. Cross-reactivity and sequence similarity between microbial transglutaminase and human antigens. *Scientific Reports*, 2023, 13:17526, doi: 10.1038/s41598-023-44452-5.

FUNCTIONAL NEUROLOGY DEFINED

Functional neurology is a branch of healthcare that focuses on understanding and optimizing the function of the nervous system, which is responsible for controlling and coordinating all the activities in our body. This discipline examines how the brain, spinal cord, and nerves work together to ensure proper communication and function. It considers the complex interactions between the parts of the nervous system and how they affect our overall health and well-being.

Functional neurology aims to promote and support the body's natural ability to heal and regulate itself. It takes a holistic approach, considering factors such as diet, lifestyle, and environmental influences impacting nervous system function. This approach can be beneficial for a wide range of conditions, including neurological disorders, chronic pain, balance and coordination problems, cognitive issues, and many others.

FUNCTIONAL MEDICINE DEFINED

Functional medicine is an approach to healthcare that focuses on identifying and addressing the root causes of disease and dysfunction in the body. Unlike traditional medicine, which often focuses on treating symptoms, functional medicine aims to understand the underlying imbalances or dysfunctions contributing to a person's health issues. It looks at the body as a whole, considering the interconnectedness of various systems and how they influence one another.

Functional medicine practitioners take a comprehensive and personalized approach to patient care. They listen to the patient's health history, symptoms, and concerns. They may use specialized testing to evaluate various aspects of their health, such as nutrient levels, hormone balance, gut health, and immune system function. Based on this information, functional medicine practitioners develop individualized treatment plans that address the underlying causes of dysfunction. Functional medicine aims to restore balance and optimize the body's natural ability to heal and function properly.

INTRODUCTION

Codes are an essential part of our daily lives. We have security codes for our homes, phones, and cars. A code aims to make critical information accessible to some people, and mysterious and untouchable to others. Codes have played significant roles in the history of our world; one excellent example is the Enigma code machine used by Nazi Germany in World War II. They used the mysterious coding machine to encrypt their top-secret messages and send them to various battlefields and battleships. It was a big part of why their "Blitzkrieg" strategy, which depended on lightning-fast movement and precise systems, was successful for so long. All the other countries thought the Enigma machine was unsolvable—except for a chosen few.

A Polish mathematician was the first person to interpret the frustrating Enigma messages. He then shared his insights with a group of determined mathematicians and scientists in England, a covert group known as Hut 6, a wartime section of the Government Code and Cypher School (GC&CS) at Bletchley Park, Buckinghamshire, United Kingdom.

This group worked for years to crack the Enigma's code. When they finally succeeded, it changed the trajectory of the war. Many historians think the Germans might have been victorious or dragged out the fight much longer if they hadn't cracked the code. Most people believed the aim of Hut 6's work was impossible, but they did it. And it changed everything.

Speaking of incredible feats that most people believed were impossible, on May 6, 1954, British runner Roger Bannister became the first person to break the four-minute mile in recorded history. Before he did it, most people thought it would never be done. Some even speculated that it was physically impossible for a human to run that fast for that long, and that the person who attempted it would probably die from exertion. On June 21, 1954, just over a month after Bannister stunned the world, John Landy became the second person to achieve a sub-four-minute mile. You see, something is only impossible until it's done. Today, a sub-four-minute mile is a standard for professional middle-distance runners.

In the same way that few people believed in the people of Hut 6's ability to break the Enigma code, or man's ability to run a sub-four minute mile, most doctors don't believe it's possible to slow, reverse, or prevent complex chronic illnesses. The top six causes of death due to chronic illness in the United States are diseases that are waging war on you, your family, and millions of other families nationwide. They are taking the lives of people we love, and we must do something about it. We can't wait for the government, Big Pharma or the so-called "experts" to figure it out. Why, you might ask? Do a Google search with the words "leading causes of death for the year 2000." You will be shocked to discover heart disease, cancer, stroke, chronic lower respiratory disease, diabetes, influenza, and Alzheimer's disease took the top spots. In over 20 years, as of writing this book, nothing has changed! It's time to move past the conventional "standard of care," which isn't working well, and consider new options. You need health practitioners willing to look outside the standard of care who read the medical research, apply what they have read, and move the needle toward "exceptional care."

You may wonder what I mean when I say the "standard of care." I'm referencing the care most hospitals or medical physicians offer and insurance companies pay for. You're not alone if you've already tried all those options and are still stuck, sick— and frustrated. If you've lost hope and are thinking, "I'll never be healed," you're probably right—if you have only received the standard of care. The United States is ranked 37th in the world in overall health care. Ouch!!! That's not very good. However, there's hope. Because beyond the standard of care is what I, and many of the doctors I've trained, offer: scientifically based, exceptional care.

There may be hope for you. If you think you've tried everything, you probably haven't. If you think there's no hope for you, look at the front and back of this book and all the testimonials in my first two books, *License to Heal* and *Highway to Health*. Those testimonials are why I'm known as the code breaker. We solve problems when all else fails. If you want to heal, you need to work with someone who has the experience and scientific backing to get the help you need.

If you're sick and tired of being sick and tired, and you want to take back your life, this book is for you. If your previous healthcare providers told you things like, "You're going to have to live with it," or "You're a professional patient," or "It's all in your head," or "You're just a chronic complainer," this book is for you.

I have been in private practice in Tupelo, Mississippi since 2001 and thousands of patients who have left hundreds of testimonials have walked through the doors of my clinic. I'm also a national and international speaker with two number-one bestselling books. Patients from 19 states and two countries have come to my clinic. I provide coaching services to a diverse range of health care professionals including chiropractors, medical doctors, PhDs, nurse practitioners and physical therapists. I have also trained doctors as far away as Spain, Dubai, and New Zealand. Now I've taken what I know about breaking the code on complex chronic illnesses and put it together in this book.

So why did I write *The Code Breaker*? Too often, when a patient's illness doesn't neatly align with insurance diagnosis codes, it is regarded as nonexistent. Maybe the patient is in a state of chronic pain and suffering, but their tissues or organs haven't been destroyed to the point at which a formal clinical diagnosis can be rendered. The patient's earnest complaints are brushed aside and labeled as a "chronic complainer," a "professional patient," a person who is only "looking for attention," or labeled as a hypochondriac, or a person suffering only from depression.

I know this may be difficult for some to accept, nevertheless it's true. All too frequently, the solution offered is a prescription for antidepressants, coupled with the suggestion to cease troubling the doctor, leaving you, the patient, with symptoms unaddressed or merely treated in isolation.

The goal of my book is to:

1. Enhance your cognitive function while improving your short- and long-term memory, organization, and multi-tasking skills.
2. Optimize your focus, attention, and concentration.
3. Sharpen your memory.
4. Improve your moBility (moving your body) and gut moTility (moving food products through your gastro-intestinal tract with proper absorption and elimination).

You may think it's impossible to slow, reverse, or even prevent these complex chronic illnesses. Still, I live in a world where people are healed daily. Even if you don't currently have a diagnosed illness, we can all use improvement in some area of our lives. There's another way to win: I'm here to help you unlock your unique and specific codes and become your own healthy and victorious code breaker.

PART ONE

UNDERSTANDING YOUR MACHINE

CHAPTER ONE

UNVEILING THE FRONTAL LOBE, THE GATEWAY TO COGNITION AND WELL-BEING

"I can accept failure, everyone fails at something. But I can't accept not trying."

—MICHAEL JORDAN

W elcome to the captivating world of the brain, where intricate neural networks shape our thoughts, emotions, and actions. In this chapter, we embark on a journey to understand the frontal lobe, an extraordinary region that holds the key to our cognitive abilities and overall well-being. The frontal lobe, with its commanding influence on cognition, autonomic function, immune responses, and gut health, stands as an extraordinary center of control within the brain. Its intricate connections and multifaceted functions highlight the interplay between the mind, body, and overall well-being. In the coming pages, we will explore the functions of the frontal lobe and its remarkable impact on the autonomic nervous system, and immune system, as well as the gut barrier and motility. Join me as we uncover the mysteries of this fascinating brain region.

THE FRONTAL LOBE AND ITS FUNCTIONS

The frontal lobe, nestled in the anterior part of the brain, is a powerhouse of cognitive functions and executive control. It orchestrates a multitude of complex processes, including reasoning, problem-solving, decision-making, and attention. Moreover, the frontal lobe plays a pivotal role in personality development, emotional regulation, and social behavior. It allows us to reason, plan for the future, and interact meaningfully with the world around us. Without the frontal lobe, our cognitive abilities and social interactions would be greatly compromised.

In addition to its role in cognition, the frontal lobe exerts a profound influence on the autonomic nervous system (ANS), which regulates essential bodily functions. The prefrontal cortex, a key region within the frontal lobe, acts as a control center, modulating the sympathetic and parasympathetic branches of the ANS. It helps maintain a delicate balance between the fight-or-flight response and rest-and-digest activities. By finely tuning the ANS, the frontal lobe contributes to our ability to adapt to stress, regulate heart rate and blood pressure, and maintain overall physiological homeostasis.

Emerging research has revealed an intriguing connection between the frontal lobe and the immune system. The frontal lobe, through its intricate network of connections with other brain regions, can influence immune responses and inflammation. It regulates the release of stress hormones, such as cortisol, which can impact immune function. Furthermore, studies suggest that the frontal lobe, particularly the prefrontal cortex, plays a role in immune cell trafficking and modulation of immune signaling molecules. This dynamic interaction between the frontal lobe and the immune system highlights the intricate relationship between the brain and overall health.

The brain-gut connection, governed in part by the frontal lobe, plays a crucial role in maintaining the integrity and function of the gastrointestinal system. The gut barrier, a complex network of cells lining the intestines, serves as the first line of defense against harmful substances. The frontal lobe, through its connection with the enteric nervous system, can influence the gut barrier's permeability and function. Additionally, the frontal lobe plays a role in regulating gut motility, ensuring the smooth movement of food through the digestive tract. Dysfunction in these processes can contribute to gastrointestinal disorders and overall well-being.

FRONTAL LOBE DEGENERATION

There are many telltale signs that show when the frontal lobe isn't healthy and thriving, which is known as frontal lobe neurodegeneration. These can occur in various neurodegenerative diseases, such as frontotemporal dementia (FTD), Alzheimer's disease, Parkinson's disease, and Huntington's disease. The signs and symptoms of frontal lobe neurodegeneration may vary depending on the specific disease and the stage of progression, but some common manifestations include:

1. Changes in personality and behavior: One of the hallmark features of frontal lobe neurodegeneration is a change in personality and behavior. Individuals may exhibit increased impulsivity, disinhibition, apathy, irritability, aggression, or inappropriate social behavior.
2. Executive dysfunction: The frontal lobe plays a crucial role in executive functions such as planning, decision-making, problem-solving, and organization. As the frontal lobe degenerates, individuals may experience difficulties with these cognitive processes, resulting in impaired judgment, poor decision-making, and decreased ability to initiate or complete tasks.

3. Language difficulties: Some individuals with frontal lobe neurodegeneration may experience language impairments, such as difficulty finding words (anomia), reduced fluency, or changes in speech patterns.

4. Motor abnormalities: In certain neurodegenerative diseases affecting the frontal lobe, individuals may experience motor abnormalities, such as muscle rigidity, tremors, or difficulty with coordination and balance.

5. Changes in social and emotional functioning: Frontal lobe neurodegeneration can lead to alterations in emotional processing and social behavior. Individuals may have difficulty recognizing or expressing emotions; they may show diminished empathy, or exhibit changes in social conduct.

6. Cognitive decline: While the primary cognitive deficits associated with frontal lobe neurodegeneration are related to executive functions, individuals may also experience impairments in attention, memory, and problem-solving abilities.

7. Personality changes: Progressive damage to the frontal lobe can result in significant changes to a person's personality. They may become more withdrawn or emotionally flattened, or they may lose interest in previously enjoyed activities.

THE PARIETAL LOBE

The parietal lobe, with its central role in sensory perception and integration, serves as a gateway to our understanding of the world around us. Its impact on the autonomic nervous system and immune system, as well as the gut barrier and motility further emphasizes the intricate relationship between the brain and overall well-being. Nestled between the frontal and occipital lobes, this remarkable region plays a vital role in sensory perception, spatial awareness, and integration of information from various senses. The parietal lobe, located towards the back of the brain, is responsible for processing and integrating sensory information from various modalities. It is divided into two primary areas: the primary somatosensory cortex and the association cortex. The primary somatosensory cortex enables us to perceive and interpret sensations, such as touch, temperature, pain, and proprioception. The association cortex integrates sensory information, allowing us to make sense of the world around us and perform complex tasks like spatial awareness, object recognition, and hand-eye coordination.

While the parietal lobe is primarily associated with sensory perception, recent studies have shed light on its impact on the autonomic nervous system (ANS). Through its connections with other brain regions, the parietal lobe can modulate ANS activity, influencing our physiological responses to external stimuli. For instance, it plays a role in regulating blood pressure, heart rate, and respiratory rate in response to sensory input. This intricate interplay between the parietal lobe and the ANS allows us to adapt to our environment and maintain homeostasis.

Studies suggest that the parietal lobe, particularly the posterior parietal cortex, can modulate immune responses. It interacts with other brain regions involved in immune regulation and influences the release of immune-signaling molecules. Additionally, the parietal lobe's role in spatial awareness and integration of sensory information may indirectly impact immune function and overall well-being.

The brain-gut connection, regulated in part by the parietal lobe, plays a crucial role in gut barrier integrity and motility. The integration of sensory information from the parietal lobe helps us perceive and respond to sensations related to digestion, such as feelings of hunger, fullness, and discomfort. Furthermore, the parietal lobe's involvement in spatial awareness and body perception may contribute to the regulation of gut motility and coordination. Dysfunction in these processes can lead to gastrointestinal disorders and affect overall gut health.

THE TEMPORAL LOBE

The temporal lobe, with its multifaceted functions, serves as a gateway to our understanding of memory, language, and auditory perception. Its impact on the autonomic nervous system, immune system, and gut barrier and motility further highlights its significant role in our overall well-being. Nestled on the sides of the cerebral cortex, the temporal lobe holds the key to various functions, including memory, language processing, and auditory perception.

The temporal lobe is a complex structure that plays a pivotal role in several cognitive functions. It encompasses the primary auditory cortex, responsible for processing sound information, and the hippocampus, vital for memory formation and consolidation. Additionally, it houses the Wernicke's area, crucial for language comprehension, and is involved in facial recognition, emotional processing, and sensory integration.

One of the most prominent functions associated with the temporal lobe is memory. The hippocampus, nestled within the temporal lobe, acts as a hub for memory formation and consolidation. It plays a crucial role in converting short-term memories into long-term memories, allowing us to retain and recall information. Damage to the temporal lobe, specifically the hippocampus, can result in memory impairments, as seen in conditions like Alzheimer's disease and temporal lobe epilepsy.

The temporal lobe's influence extends beyond memory, reaching into the realm of autonomic nervous system (ANS) regulation. Through its connections with other brain regions, the temporal lobe can modulate ANS activity, impacting physiological responses to various stimuli. For example, it plays a role in emotional processing and can influence heart rate, blood pressure, and respiration. These connections highlight the temporal lobe's involvement in the body's visceral responses and emotional regulation.

While the temporal lobe's impact on the immune system is not as extensively studied as other functions, there is evidence to suggest its involvement. The temporal lobe, particularly the amygdala and hippocampus, interacts with brain regions involved in immune regulation. This interaction can influence the release of immune-signaling molecules and modulate immune responses.

The temporal lobe's involvement in sensory integration and emotional processing may indirectly affect gut function. Emotional states, processed within the temporal lobe, have been known to impact gut motility and barrier integrity. Moreover, disruptions in the temporal lobe, such as in individuals with temporal lobe epilepsy, have been associated with gastrointestinal symptoms.

THE OCCIPITAL LOBE

The occipital lobe, situated at the back of the cerebral cortex, serves as the gateway to visual perception and understanding. Its intricate functions not only encompass visual processing but also extend to memory formation, autonomic nervous system regulation, and potential impacts on the immune system and gut function. The occipital lobe is primarily responsible for visual processing, acting as the brain's visual powerhouse. It contains the primary visual cortex, where incoming visual stimuli from the eyes are transformed into meaningful images. The occipital lobe also houses higher-order visual association areas, which help us recognize objects and faces, and to navigate our visual environment.

While the occipital lobe's primary function is vision, it also has a subtle impact on memory formation and retrieval. Visual stimuli are essential in encoding memories, and the occipital lobe plays a crucial role in this process. By processing and interpreting visual information, the occipital lobe contributes to the formation of vivid and detailed memories. Additionally, damage can result in visual memory impairments, affecting an individual's ability to recall visual details.

The occipital lobe's influence extends beyond vision, reaching into the realm of the autonomic nervous system (ANS). Visual stimuli processed by the occipital lobe can trigger autonomic responses, such as changes in heart rate, blood pressure, and respiratory rate. For example, witnessing a frightening or beautiful scene can evoke emotional responses that modulate ANS activity. These connections highlight the occipital lobe's involvement in our physiological responses to visual stimuli.

While the occipital lobe's direct impact on the immune system is not extensively studied, its role in visual perception indirectly influences immune responses. Visual stimuli, processed within the occipital lobe, can trigger emotional responses that, in turn, modulate immune function. The emotional experiences associated with visual stimuli can influence the release of immune-signaling molecules and impact immune responses.

THE CEREBELLUM

The cerebellum, often overshadowed by its larger counterparts, plays a crucial role in motor coordination, balance, and posture. Beyond its motor functions, the cerebellum contributes to memory formation, influences the autonomic nervous system, and potentially impacts the immune system and gut barrier and motility. Nestled beneath the cerebral cortex, the cerebellum is often associated with motor coordination. However, its influence extends far beyond that.

The cerebellum, often referred to as the "little brain," is responsible for coordinating voluntary movements and maintaining balance and posture. It receives inputs from various sensory systems and integrates them with motor signals from the cerebral cortex to fine-tune movements. Additionally, the cerebellum plays a role in cognitive functions, such as attention, language, and executive functions.

While memory is traditionally associated with the hippocampus and other cortical regions, recent research suggests the cerebellum's involvement in certain forms of memory. It is particularly implicated in motor learning and procedural memory, which involve acquiring and retaining skills and habits.

The cerebellum's ability to adapt and refine movements over time contributes to the formation and retrieval of motor memories.

Although primarily known for its role in motor coordination, the cerebellum also exerts an influence on the autonomic nervous system (ANS). Through connections with brainstem nuclei involved in autonomic regulation, the cerebellum modulates ANS activity. This influence can manifest in various ways, such as regulating heart rate, blood pressure, and respiratory rhythm. The cerebellum's involvement in the ANS highlights its integrative nature within the broader neural network.

While the direct impact of the cerebellum on the immune system is not extensively studied, emerging evidence suggests its involvement in immune regulation. The cerebellum receives inputs from regions involved in immune responses, including the brainstem and prefrontal cortex. These connections provide a potential avenue for the cerebellum to modulate immune function.

The cerebellum's influence on the gut barrier and motility is an area of ongoing investigation. While direct connections between the cerebellum and gut function are limited, emerging evidence suggests that the cerebellum may indirectly influence gut health. Its role in coordinating movements and maintaining balance may impact gut motility. Additionally, its involvement in cognitive functions could influence gut-brain interactions, potentially impacting gut barrier integrity.

THE GUT: THE SECOND BRAIN

The gut, often referred to as the second brain, plays a significant role in our physical and mental health. Its complex network of

neurons, known as the enteric nervous system, allows it to function independently and communicate bidirectionally with the
brain. The human body is a complex and fascinating organism,
with various organs and systems working together to ensure our
overall well-being. When discussing the gut, it is often referred
to as the "second brain" due to its intricate connection with the
central nervous system and its significant impact on our physical
and mental health.

The gastrointestinal tract is a long tube-like structure that
begins at the mouth and ends at the anus. It consists of several
organs, including the esophagus, stomach, small intestine, large
intestine, and rectum. The gut is responsible for the digestion
and absorption of nutrients from the food we consume, as well
as the elimination of waste materials.

The term "second brain" is often used to describe the extensive network of nerves present in the gut, known as the enteric
nervous system (ENS). The ENS is composed of millions of
neurons that are embedded in the walls of the digestive tract,
extending from the esophagus to the rectum. This intricate
network allows the gut to function independently of the central
nervous system (CNS) in the brain.

The gut and the brain communicate bidirectionally through
multiple pathways, forming what is known as the gut-brain axis.
The ENS can send signals to the brain, influencing our emotions, mood, and overall mental state. Similarly, the brain can
send signals to the gut, affecting digestion, gut motility, and the
release of hormones and neurotransmitters.

Notably, the gut produces a wide range of neurotransmitters,
including serotonin, dopamine, and gamma-aminobutyric acid
(GABA), which are also found in the brain. Serotonin, for example,
plays a crucial role in regulating mood, and approximately 90% of

serotonin in the body is produced in the gut. This highlights the significance of the gut-brain axis in mental health and well-being.

Research has shown that the gut's health and its communication with the brain have a profound impact on various aspects of our overall health. Imbalances in gut bacteria, known as dysbiosis, have been linked to various conditions such as irritable bowel syndrome (IBS), inflammatory bowel disease (IBD), obesity, and even mental health disorders like depression and anxiety.

Furthermore, studies have demonstrated that gut health may influence immune function, skin health, and even cognitive abilities. Maintaining a healthy gut through a balanced diet, regular exercise, and stress management techniques is crucial for optimizing overall health and well-being.

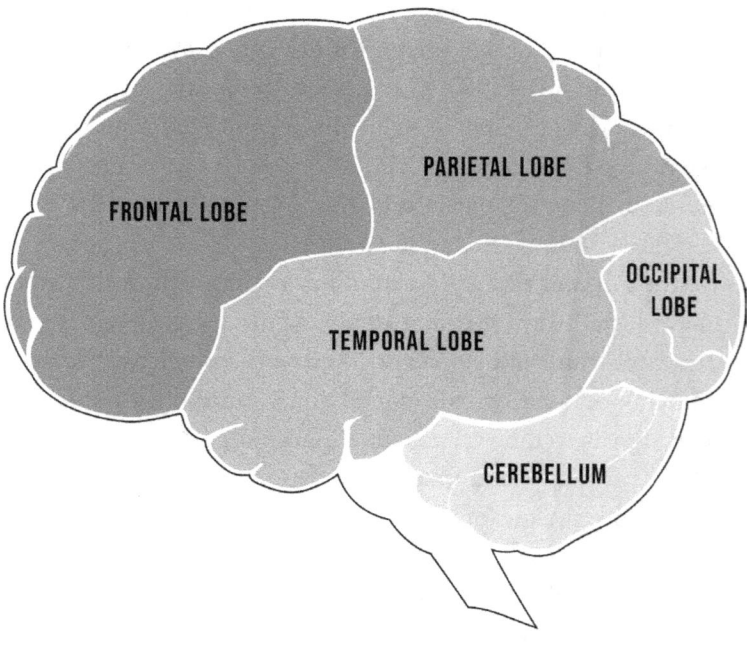

Below is a case study submitted by one of my Barlow Brain and Body Institute students, Dr. Bryce Cunningham D.C., C.C.S.T. This story exemplifies why we must address inflammation in the brain and gut simultaneously to achieve optimal results.

****

A 77-year-old male patient came to me exhibiting eight years of fatigue and vertigo and starting to show signs of mild cognitive impairment with short- and long-term memory loss. He admitted to staying in bed longer than usual before getting up and starting his day. He also had to take naps to make it through the day. Along with being unstable and foggy-headed, his vision had changed, and he couldn't get any glasses that helped.

This patient couldn't handle riding in a car when someone else was driving. It made him feel sick and worsened his vertigo. Usually, he had to lie down and nap to recover. This significantly interfered with his life and hobbies. Stress also made his symptoms worse. Things that caused even small amounts of stress made his symptoms worsen. He had been to nine doctors and "specialists." With no results or answers, he had almost given up hope for any help.

Upon evaluation, he presented with mild sensory deficits in the lower extremities and decreased cerebellar function, which resulted in poor coordination of movement for the upper and lower extremities. Assessment of his eye movements revealed anterior and posterior canal deficits.

I prescribed a 10-week gut, brain, and liver detox. A blood chemistry lab of 77 markers was ordered, along with Cyrex lab panels #2, #3, #4, #5, #11, #12, and Alzheimer's L.I.N.X.

At-home neurological therapy was prescribed to include the infra-red plate and nerve plate. This therapy increased blood flow to the extremities and exercised nerve pathways. Infra-red ultrabright was also used to increase blood flow to the lobes of the brain.

Within a week of starting the detox, his neighbors, who didn't even know he was getting treatment, could tell the difference in his activity levels. Once the blood work returned and revealed what was driving his decline in function and overall enjoyment of life, we made lifestyle changes to help him avoid those factors.

A year later, he reports much-improved energy and stamina. He is waking up and starting his day about two hours earlier than when he was struggling. Memory and recall have returned. Riding in the car when someone else is driving has improved, and he can travel for several hours to see family. According to his wife, his character and personality have returned. He says it's because he's not constantly feeling sick and dizzy. Now he is returning to the activities and hobbies he had previously given up. Some things he is doing now that would not have been possible before treatment include golfing, riding in a car for several hours, working around his house, repairing a wooden deck, hunting, fishing, and having an addition built onto his home. Oh, and by the way, he just had a check-up with his eye doctor, and his vision is now 20/20 again! He doesn't need to wear glasses every day.

Dr. Bryce Cunningham
Round Rock, Texas

Are you hungry for more insights?
Visit www.thecodebreakeronline.com for an even
deeper dive into the subjects covered in this chapter.

CHAPTER TWO

THE POWER OF A CODE

"Do one thing every day that scares you"

—ELEANOR ROOSEVELT

magine we're having lunch together, and I hand you my locked iPhone. Do you think you could enter the correct code to unlock it? Probably not. Could you enter your own phone's code and unlock it? Again, probably not. Your code won't work on my phone, and my code won't work on your phone. Even though our phones may look the same, the same code doesn't unlock the two phones.

However, if I gave you the code to my phone, unlocking it would be a much easier process. Similar to the iPhone example above, a person's chronic illness possesses a unique multivariate neuro-metabolic code that must be broken so they can heal. This neuro-metabolic code cannot be broken using the conventional "standard of care" method. The key to deciphering it lies in conducting a comprehensive neurological examination and doing extensive metabolic testing. Remember, "If we don't test, it's only a guess."

Perhaps you haven't considered that there are specific codes that can unlock the mysteries of your chronic health problems. This is one of the reasons I wrote this book: to reveal these codes, assist you in unlocking them, and give you the life you want and deserve. Through my years in practice and doing extensive research, I've discovered there are seven metabolic factors, seven "codes," if you will, that contribute, in varying degrees, to the development and progression of complex chronic illnesses like Alzheimer's disease, Parkinson's disease, multiple sclerosis, and many more. In the coming chapters, I will provide clear, understandable explanations as we delve deeply into each of the seven codes. By decoding these factors and removing the triggers, your body gains a greater chance to heal.

An important aspect of interpreting your body's seven codes is bloodwork. Specific metabolic tests help identify the codes that require unlocking to address your body's health issues. These tests unveil your body's unique triggers and whether they stem from genetics, environmental factors, or a breach in your gut and/or brain barrier systems. Once we know these triggers, we use the four Rs to optimize your recovery:

1. Remove: Detox the brain, body, and gut.
2. Repair and Restore: Unlock your specific codes through up to 10 lab tests.
3. Regenerate—the brain, body, and gut by activating deficient pathways. Create neuroplasticity, which forms new pathways between the brain, body, and gut.

SOLVING THE PUZZLE

Have you ever had a repairman come to your house? Say you have termite damage or mold in one of your walls. The handyman will probably tell you that you need to remove the damaged and moldy materials, i.e., remove the triggers causing the damage, and then replace the wall. Well, I often joke that I'm in the body reconstruction business. Instead of using hammers and drills, I use blood tests, the latest scientific research, and advanced therapies to generate extraordinary results for you and your family.

Each code we investigate is akin to a tree, and just as a tree has numerous branches, these seven codes may also branch into various sub-codes. It takes a lot of Sherlock Holmes-style work to determine the major codes and sub-codes that are working together to cause your health problems. However, these exceptional care strategies have changed bloodwork results, reduced or eliminated chronic pain, reversed cognitive decline and movement disorders, and given people their lives and freedom. So what are we doing that's so different? How are we reversing these complex chronic illnesses?

Right now, I have the latest iPhone. It's current and up to date, but guess what? It'll be outdated in five years. The same is true with medical research. The latest papers and medical journals constantly reveal new insights into the origins of these complex chronic illnesses, including methods for early trigger identification and appropriate intervention.

It's peculiar that we eagerly seek the latest and most advanced technology for our phones, TVs, and cars, yet we seem content with a "standard of care" healthcare model that hasn't significantly evolved since the 1980s: difficult to comprehend, nevertheless true. Name one chronic disease eradicated in the past 40 years. I'll wait—because there isn't one! The "standard of care" hasn't changed much in four decades. Today, more people than ever suffer from heart disease, cancer, chronic lower respiratory disease, stroke, Alzheimer's, and diabetes as they did in the 1980s, 1990s, and 2000s. It appears that the conventional healthcare system, often called the "standard of care," offers only limited solutions for individuals facing these challenges.

I'm a voracious learner who wakes up at 4:00 a.m. each morning to read the latest research journals. My team and I are passionate about what we do, leaving no stone unturned in our relentless quest to address our patients' conditions. I wish the standards for healthcare matched the advancements in Silicon Valley technology. Silicon Valley is renowned for pushing the boundaries of technological innovation. It has consistently set the pace for advancement from smartphones to self-driving cars. However, our "standard of care" healthcare system lags behind.

I'm asking: Why can't healthcare be as innovative as consumer technology? My answer: It can be and is, but it can't be found in the "standard of care" model. The key is identifying your unique combination of codes and then minimizing or altogether avoiding them. Once we do that, we can improve, slow down, and restore function. You can find hope. You may be one appointment away from a significant shift in your life!

UNDERSTANDING ALZHEIMER'S

America's top six chronic illnesses are cardiovascular disease, cancer, chronic lower respiratory disease, stroke, Alzheimer's, and diabetes. Alzheimer's, also known to many people as "dementia," has four early warning signs that are frequently ignored or scoffed at by individuals, their family members, and even their healthcare providers:

1. Loss of endurance (mental and physical)
2. Loss of focus
3. Loss of attention
4. Loss of concentration

These symptoms are often lumped together and called "brain fog." Do you walk into a room and forget why? Do you ever call someone and can't remember why? Do you ever get lost in conversation? Some laugh off these symptoms with casual jokes like, "Getting older sucks," or "I have the mind of an 80-year-old." I encourage you to take these early warning signs seriously. If you had a large gash on your leg, you'd go to a doctor for an exam and stitches. In the same way, take these mental symptoms seriously. These are all red flags, warning signs of cognitive decline, as well as a golden opportunity to slow down or possibly reverse the damage. Although these early warning signs give the person the best opportunity for recovery, most will roll their eyes, shrug their shoulders, laugh it off and do nothing about it. Others, however, will take a more proactive approach, heed these early warning signs and change their lives.

Currently, research predicts that global dementia will triple by 2050. In America, six million people have Alzheimer's disease. One in nine is aged under 65, and two-thirds of all people diagnosed with Alzheimer's are women. And this number will triple in just three decades? That's a severe problem.

Do you know when the first person was diagnosed with Alzheimer's disease? Alzheimer's got its name from a German psychiatrist and neuropathologist, Dr. Alois Alzheimer. On November 3, 1906 in Frankfurt, Germany, Dr. Alzheimer noticed changes in the brain tissue of a woman who had died of an unusual mental illness. Her name was Auguste Deter. Her symptoms included memory loss, language problems, and unpredictable behavior. We've gone from the first person diagnosed in 1906 to over six million Americans diagnosed with Alzheimer's disease in 2023. Take a minute to reflect on the significant impact of those numbers and the rapid progression of the disease. Henry Ford was once quoted as saying, "If you always do what you always did, you'll always get what you always got."

Looking at those statistics, I believe that's Western medicine's way of saying, "We don't have an answer for this." To bring this point home even further, one-in-six people in the United States currently have a neurological disorder, the top ones being headaches, multiple sclerosis, dementia, stroke, and Parkinson's.

Dementia is an umbrella term for several diseases affecting memory, cognitive abilities, and behavior, which all interfere significantly with a person's ability to maintain activities of daily living. The four most common types of dementia are: 1) Alzheimer's disease. The most common form of dementia representing 60–80% of all dementia diagnoses 2) vascular dementia 3) frontotemporal dementia and 4) Lewy body dementia.

These diseases are like an 18-wheeler: They start slowly but quickly gain speed and momentum. Your ability to focus, maintain attention, and concentrate, along with personality changes, are among the first aspects to be impacted by the disease. Our daily habits and lifestyle choices, most of which we are completely unaware of, have a significant impact on the rate at which our brain may degenerate. By adopting certain lifestyle practices, we can slow down this process and maintain better cognitive health.

The problem with Alzheimer's disease, as well as other complex chronic illnesses which are discussed in this book, is that it's a multivariate problem. Multiple things we do wrong, like poor diet or lifestyle habits, compound across the decades to cause this disease. Bottom line: our daily habits, diet, and lifestyle choices play a crucial role in our brain health over time.

Our dietary choices, which will be covered in depth in The Code Breaker, significantly impact our healing and recovery process, as well as our overall health trajectory. The speed at which we heal and whether we experience a decline in health largely depends on what we consume. Eating a nutritionally balanced diet is crucial for effectively slowing down, reversing, and preventing complex chronic illnesses. Equally important is how well we absorb nutrients into our bloodstream. Making informed decisions about our food intake is paramount in promoting optimal health outcomes. Consuming a diverse range of nutrient-dense foods, including fruits, vegetables, lean proteins, and healthy fats, provides the essential nutrients our bodies need to function optimally.

In this era of Big Pharma and constant advertising of prescription drugs, why isn't there an answer for Alzheimer's? The 2019 Frontiers in Human Neuroscience publication trends report showed a total of 181,116 articles regarding Alzheimer's disease. According to StandfordHealthcare.org there are only three FDA-approved drugs to treat the symptoms of mild-to-moderate Alzheimer's disease. While these drugs may delay decline in memory and reduce confusion, they are not curative and are unable to stop the disease from worsening over time. Hmm, 181,116 articles and only three drugs to treat mild-to-moderate symptoms, wow! We have three drugs trying to have a positive impact on a person suffering from a multivariant health issue. Clearly, that approach isn't working.

Starting in 2013, scientists increasingly recognized Alzheimer's as a disease process that begins years before symptoms of dementia become evident. Now, new research has found changes in the brain and body up to 20 years before Alzheimer's symptoms arise. The study identified elevated levels of beta-amyloid, a toxic protein that builds up in the brains of those with Alzheimer's. They found that brain plaques, a hallmark of Alzheimer's, begin 15 years before memory problems become evident.

Now, let's fast-forward from 2013 to the present day. Wouldn't it be great if we could test for predictive antibodies to amyloid-beta and tau proteins? Spoiler alert: we can! It's the Cyrex Alzheimer's LINX blood test. But you see, these tests aren't your "standard of care" tests. Unfortunately, the standard of care is a wait-and-see game. "Let's wait and see what happens." Meanwhile your brain continues to degenerate.

So why doesn't a simple, magical silver bullet heal dementia? Think of a complex chronic illness like a pan of homemade, gluten-free lasagna. What's in lasagna? Well, lots of things. Cheese, meat, noodles, sauce, and more. It takes many ingredients. If you only put cheese in the pan and then put it in the oven, you don't get lasagna; you get melted cheese. The same is true with complex chronic illnesses. You can't expect one silver bullet, one magical drug, or one type of therapy to slow down, prevent or reverse the issue because it's multivariate. The solution will require a multimodal approach with both neurological and metabolic interventions.

When it comes to slowing or preventing a complex chronic illness like Alzheimer's disease, time is of the essence. There are seven stages of the disease, and once you reach stage five and beyond, I can no longer accept you for care at my clinic. You are too advanced to make any meaningful impact on your life. If you or your loved one is in stages one through four, help maybe available.

THE SEVEN STAGES OF ALZHEIMER'S

Stage One: No cognitive decline

Stage Two: Mild decline, very occasional forgetfulness. You may be the only one who notices these changes at this stage, also known as subjective cognitive impairment (SCI). At this stage, only you can tell something is cognitively "off." You know your focus, attention, and concentration are slipping.

Stage Three: Focus, attention, concentration, and brain fog problems occasionally, once to twice a month. This is when other people start noticing something is amiss.

Stage Four: This is everyday brain fog. Stages three and four are considered Mild Cognitive Impairment (MCI). This name is actually oxymoronic because it's like saying, "I have mild metastatic cancer."

In stages two to four, the patient says, "I'm unable to focus as well as I did in the past. I need help; something is wrong." Yet, family, friends, and doctors tell them everything is perfectly fine. "You're just getting older." "No, my brain fog is getting worse," the patient insists. They get the same response, "This is a normal part of aging." Then, you can't remember where you parked your car at the store. Now, you know something is terribly wrong, but still, no one will listen.

Stage Five: Things take a dramatic turn at stage five. At this point, the person has so much neuroinflammation and neurodegeneration that they no longer see themselves as the problem. They become cognitively rigid with a "my way or the highway attitude." He or she starts blaming others and wants to know why their spouse keeps "hiding" the TV remote, cell phone, or coffee mug. The person may no longer bathe or brush their teeth. Hygiene is of little importance to the person in stages five, six and seven.

This person has been begging for help for the past 20 years, and everyone laughed it off, rolled their eyes, shrugged their shoulders, and blamed it on age. Finally, when everyone is serious about improving the family member's health, the family member isn't. Why? Because they're in stage five and no longer see themselves as having a problem. Now, everyone else is the problem. Unfortunately, it's now too late. No one listened in stages two through four; now nothing can be done to improve cognitive function.

I understand that all this information is eye-opening and can feel overwhelming. Please keep reading and remain open to the truth in these pages. Knowing all this information is like being in the Matrix; you can choose the blue pill, bury your head in the sand, and keep going down the same path. Or you can choose the red pill, wake up to the truth in front of you, and see the situation as it is. I am, and forever will be, Team Red Pill. We each have to take responsibility for our lives and the quality thereof.

Your health should be such that you can do whatever you want. Is that traveling? Spending time with your family? Golfing? In my case, it's racquetball. Whatever it is, you must take responsibility for your health situation. Seek beyond the standard of care because it will never give you the exceptional life you deserve. Remember, there is "standard of care" and there is "exceptional care." It's your life. It's your choice.

Are you hungry for more insights?
Visit www.thecodebreakeronline.com for an even
deeper dive into the subjects covered in this chapter.

CHAPTER THREE

REDUCTIONISM VS. HOLISM

"Always do your best. What you plant now, will harvest later."

—OG MANDINO

When solving a complex issue like chronic illness, we look at potential solutions to the problem matters. There are two kinds of "lenses" that health practitioners wear when working with a patient. The first is worn by many traditional healthcare professionals (and some scientific researchers), and is known as "reductionism." The reductionist approach in healthcare means that doctors and scientists try to understand and treat health problems by studying and focusing on smaller, specific parts of the body. People wearing this set of lenses believe they can figure out exactly how the body works and what particular things cause diseases. This approach wants to boil the problem and the solution down to one cause and one cure.

Reductionism seeks to understand and explain complex biological, physiological, and pathological phenomena by breaking them into smaller, simpler components or parts. This reductionist approach focuses on studying and analyzing individual elements, such as genes, molecules, cells, or specific physiological functions, believing that understanding these smaller parts will lead to a comprehensive understanding of the whole system or disease process.

The reductionist approach helps us understand the intricate details of biological processes, diseases, and treatments at a molecular and cellular level. By breaking things down into smaller components, we gain detailed insight into specific mechanisms and can develop targeted interventions. This reductionist knowledge forms the foundation for medical science.

On the other hand, some practitioners primarily wear a second set of lenses, known as "holism." Holistic healthcare takes a more comprehensive approach, looking at your overall well-being and considering many things that can affect your health. It recognizes that many interconnected factors influence your health and well-being, including physical, mental, emotional, social, diet and environmental aspects. Holistic healthcare considers the person as a whole rather than focusing solely on specific symptoms or diseases. It acknowledges the intricate interplay between various dimensions of an individual's life and seeks to promote balance and harmony. By considering the whole person and their unique circumstances, holistic healthcare can address the underlying causes and promote overall well-being. It emphasizes the importance of lifestyle, nutrition, and mental health in maintaining health and preventing diseases.

THE BEST OF BOTH

Almost all healthcare professionals are of the reductionist mindset, and holism is the opposite of reductionism. Here's what makes me unique from most doctors: I wear both sets of lenses simultaneously. We need both reductionist and holistic approaches in healthcare because they offer complementary perspectives and strengths that can broaden our understanding and treatment of complex chronic diseases.

Integrating reductionist and holistic approaches allows for personalized, tailored, and exceptional care. Reductionist approaches help identify specific factors or mechanisms contributing to a patient's symptoms. In contrast, holistic approaches consider the broader context and individual needs, diet, environmental triggers, and gastrointestinal health, as well as cognitive health. By combining these perspectives, healthcare providers can develop effective and considerate treatment plans for the patient's well-being.

Reductionist and holistic approaches often complement each other. Reductionist research and discoveries contribute to the development of new treatments and interventions. Holistic approaches, on the other hand, can improve patient outcomes by addressing the underlying causes, promoting self-care, and enhancing overall quality of life.

Healthcare is a complex field, and no single approach can capture its entirety. By combining reductionist and holistic perspectives, healthcare professionals can tackle the complexity of human health more effectively. It allows us to balance the detailed understanding of specific processes at the cellular level, with the broader context of the patient's life and health, while looking at diet and lifestyle, as well as the environment in which we live.

Integrating reductionist and holistic approaches in healthcare allows us to combine detailed scientific knowledge at the micro level with a comprehensive understanding of the whole person: the macro level. This synergistic approach enhances our ability to provide personalized, effective, and patient-centered care, ultimately serving patients in an exceptional manner that helps them gain real, lasting, and meaningful results.

GOING BEYOND THE "STANDARD"

I was excited when I bought my first home. I thought it was a great house, and it was. But there was one problem: A leaky pipe under the sink left me with a surprise and an unsightly hole in my kitchen wall underneath the sink. I called a professional to come out and tell me what it would cost to fix the hole. When he told me that the wall, my cabinets, and half of the kitchen floor needed to be replaced, what I thought would be a simple patch job turned into a major renovation project. He needed to start from solid wood and rebuild. I saw a hole, but he saw rot and water damage that extended several feet from the source of the leak. I did what was needed. I had the contractor fix the walls, cabinets, and floor because I knew that if I didn't fully fix the problem, I'd have bigger issues.

The hole in my kitchen floor was similar to a "check engine" light on a car. The light flashes on the dash, indicating that there's a problem. While the blinking engine light doesn't provide precise details, it serves as a vital warning, indicating something is wrong and demands our attention. Putting duct tape over the blinking light may cover up the symptom, but it doesn't fix the problem. Covering up your health symptoms and not addressing root causes is analogous to duct tape on a blinking engine light.

Patients walking through my clinic door usually have had multiple years of "blinky lights" on their "dashboard" of health. They've been to every traditional Western medicine doctor they could think of and have been told time and again to accept their condition and "learn to live with it." These patients usually use multiple prescription medications to manage their blinky light symptoms because doctors are trained in a reductionist mindset to focus on the idea of one symptom, one drug: five symptoms, five drugs. You probably know a family member or friend who is currently living that life. That's why the traditional medical system has failed them. The system treats the symptoms not the cause. There's no interaction between doctor and patient about diet or lifestyle choices, just, "here's your prescription and see you next time."

Reductionism is exceptional at treating acute problems. For example, if you have a sore throat, you may go to the doctor, get swabbed, and learn you have strep throat. You take an antibiotic that kills the infectious bacteria and you are good to go. That's a good application of reductionist medicine.

The approach has to change when we go from acute to multivariate, chronic care. Most healthcare professionals are trained to be reductionists. This is why modern medical practices often prescribe a single pill to alleviate a specific symptom rather than considering the holistic health of the entire body. When you look at things from a reductionist standpoint, you try to find the one thing to make the blinky light disappear.

When solving complex chronic illnesses, you can't just be a holist or reductionist; you must marry the two for the patient's best interest. I use both views and both pairs of lenses when needed. One is not better than the other. We need both to find and untangle the root causes of chronic issues. There's more going on in there than a simple, single problem Here's an example of one of my patients. His primary complaint was numbness and tingling in his feet. His secondary complaint was bloating and constipation. After a little digging, I learned he also had anxiety issues and insomnia.

I performed a neurological exam and recommended he do all the metabolic tests. We found inflammation levels through the roof, insulin resistance, leaky gut, leaky brain, gluten and casein sensitivity, dental bacteria, and two rouge bacteria in his gastrointestinal tract. I referred him to a local nurse practitioner and a local dentist. Solving these complex chronic illnesses is a team sport; you need team players. We used both approaches: the reductionist approach via the nurse practitioner and dentist, and the holistic approach via me. As you can see there are many factors at play. It is truly a web of physiological dysfunction. The "blinky light syndrome" approach to treating the symptom works great for acute health problems. However, it has been an abysmal failure in addressing and correcting complex chronic illnesses. But you don't have to believe me; just look at the research. As I stated earlier, America is ranked 37th in the world in overall health. Don't make me pull out the Henry Ford quote again.

My approach is unique as I conduct a comprehensive, head-to-toe neurological exam and utilize cutting-edge laboratories, like Cyrex Labs, to isolate specific metabolic triggers. These are the steps I follow to be "The Code Breaker." We give you exceptional care and leave no stone unturned. We must look at the overall body, do the work, and find the triggers of these multivariate, complex chronic health problems because, as most of us know, the current "standard of care" system isn't working. Instead of "standard of care," we use the latest scientific research to apply it to your life and body.

Are you hungry for more insights?
Visit www.thecodebreakeronline.com for an even
deeper dive into the subjects covered in this chapter.

PART TWO

UNDERSTANDING THE CODES

CHAPTER FOUR

THE SEVEN CODES: AN INTRODUCTION

"Sometimes, when you think things are falling apart, they may actually be falling into place."

—Unknown

As we learn more about the seven codes, including what they are, how they affect our health, how to identify them, and what to do about them, we must understand that we all have a unique "web of psychological dysfunction." In the coming chapters, we'll learn about the codes individually, but no one has just one code that needs to be broken. It's more like a toxic soup. What's in vegetable soup? Many kinds of vegetables in varying ratios. What's in your unique web of dysfunction? Many codes, in varying degrees, are presented in unique ways.

There are pages and pages of research saying that if you have just one of these codes, it's enough to cause systemic inflammation, leaky gut, leaky brain, neuroinflammation, brain fog, and neurodegeneration. But what happens if you have two different codes, maybe three, four, or five of them? You need someone to walk you through unpacking your codes and unwinding their tangled web. In this book—and in my clinic—that's exactly what I help my readers and patients do. We examine the symptoms and the whole picture of each person's health to crack the codes and get results. From a holistic standpoint, we look at everything, never taking any portion of your life or health journey off the table so that we can crack your codes and help you achieve vibrant health and radiant energy. Now, let's look at a summary of each code and how it may show up in your life.

CODE #1 INFLAMMATION

There are two types of inflammation: acute and chronic. Acute inflammation happens when you sprain your ankle, which becomes swollen and is hot to the touch, red, and painful. The body has an inflammatory response to an injury, which triggers the start of the healing process. Chronic, or systemic, inflammation is like an out-of-control wildfire inside your body that can harm your brain, body, and gut. It is associated with an increased risk of various chronic conditions, including cardiovascular disease, type 2 diabetes, autoimmune disorders, neurodegenerative diseases, gastrointestinal disorders, cognitive decline, mood disorders, and an increased risk of neurodegenerative diseases such as Alzheimer's and Parkinson's. These issues all link to chronic inflammation in the brain. Chronic inflammation contributes to tissue damage, organ dysfunction, and an increased risk of chronic diseases in the body. In the gut, it can disrupt the balance of gut microbiota, impair nutrient absorption, and contribute to conditions like inflammatory bowel disease (IBD).

CODE #2 BLOOD SUGAR DYSREGULATION

Blood sugar is to the body as gasoline is to a car. It's the fuel for powering the mitochondria. Think of the mitochondria as a nuclear power plant inside our cells. Your mitochondria need glucose (octane) and oxygen to run optimally; just as your car has an optimal range for octane to perform perfectly, your blood sugar also has an optimal range of 85–99 and an A1C below 5.3. These two numbers are crucial for maintaining the overall health and functioning of the brain, body, and gut. When blood sugar levels are consistently too high (above 99) or too low (below 85), it can have devastating effects on the mitochondria, brain, body, and gut.

CODE #3 MALABSORPTION ISSUES

The major player here is called "leaky gut." Malabsorption and leaky gut refer to the impaired absorption of nutrients from the gastrointestinal tract into the bloodstream. This condition can devastate the human brain, body, and gut, depriving the body of essential nutrients, minerals, amino acids, carbohydrates, and healthy fats needed for optimal functioning. It leads to an inability to draw the nutrition from our food to give our body the building blocks and raw materials it needs to heal. Also with leaky gut, undigested proteins and bacteria can leak out of the gut into the sterile bloodstream, leading to chronic inflammation and an over-aroused immune system.

CODE #4 PATHOGENS AND TOXIC OVERLOAD

This code refers to the toxic overload our body receives from living in a contaminated world. Unfortunately, environmental toxins are everywhere, including in plastics, cleaning supplies, herbicides, pesticides, makeup, and paints. According to the CDC website, we're exposed to over 700,000 toxins daily.

I know that sounds overwhelming, but when we focus on cracking this code, we aim to eliminate the most significant risk factors like mold, dental pathogens and heavy metals, and more. The healthier your body gets, the better it can handle small exposures to other obscure toxins. The most critical part of solving this code is using lab tests like Cyrex array #11 and #12 to identify the toxins that trigger your body's negative response. Once we know the triggers, we can minimize exposure or remove them altogether from your life.

CODE #5 AUTOIMMUNE DISORDERS

This code of autoimmune disease happens when the body's natural defense, our immune system, can't tell the difference between your cells and foreign cells, called antigens (antigens could be gluten, casein, mold, viruses, bacteria and many more), mistakenly causing the body to attack normal cells. Autoimmune disorders are examples of "friendly fire" happening to our body as the immune system goes into overdrive, attacking our own body's organs and tissues. More than 80 types of autoimmune diseases may affect many body parts. Cyrex Labs array #5 is a predictive antibody test in which the immune system tags your body's organs and tissues for destruction.

CODE #6 TRAUMA (PHYSICAL, MENTAL, EMOTIONAL, PTSD)

The trauma code can involve either physical and/or mental/ emotional trauma. Physical trauma would include harm caused to the body due to accidents, violence, or other external forces. Emotional trauma, conversely, pertains to the psychological impact of distressing events that overwhelm our ability to cope effectively. It could result from abuse, loss of a loved one, or witnessing violence, leading to symptoms like anxiety, depression, and trouble forming healthy relationships. The brain doesn't make a significant distinction between physical and emotional trauma, which means the death of a loved one could have nearly as much physical impact on your brain, body, and gut as a car accident. The key to solving this code is identifying the source of the trauma and then unwinding the web of dysfunction it has caused.

CODE #7 VASCULAR ISSUES

High blood pressure (hypertension) and low blood pressure (hypotension) are two common conditions that affect blood flow and can contribute to complex chronic illnesses differently. High blood pressure occurs when the force of blood against the artery walls is consistently too high. This pressure strains the heart and blood vessels, leading to potential damage over time. Hypertension is often asymptomatic, earning it the nickname "the silent killer." Low blood pressure leads to reduced blood flow to vital organs. Common symptoms may include dizziness, fainting, fatigue, and blurry vision. While mild hypotension is generally not a cause for concern, severe or chronic low blood pressure can lead to complications like inadequate blood supply to the brain, heart, and other organs. Addressing the root cause and managing low blood pressure is crucial to preventing complications and related chronic diseases. The main symptom of these kinds of vascular issues is cold hands and feet, which almost always means the brain isn't getting enough blood as well.

The journey to becoming a code breaker and solving complex chronic illnesses means understanding the seven major codes that contribute to the web of dysfunction, which can lead to complex chronic diseases. Each code presents a unique, complex puzzle, from addressing inflammation, blood sugar dysregulation, and malabsorption issues to tackling pathogens, toxic overload, vascular problems, autoimmune disorders, and trauma. By unraveling and understanding the interconnectedness of these factors, we can devise comprehensive treatment plans that target the root causes of your struggles. Combining evidence-based therapies, lifestyle modifications, and personalized approaches, we can pave the way toward improved health, enhanced well-being, and a brighter future for those battling complex chronic illnesses. Let's spend the following chapters digging into each code individually.

Are you hungry for more insights?
Visit www.thecodebreakeronline.com for an even deeper dive into the subjects covered in this chapter.

CHAPTER FIVE

CODE #1 CHRONIC INFLAMMATION

"You're braver than you believe, stronger than
you seem, and smarter than you think."

—A.A. MILNE

There's a difference between a fire that burns merrily inside a fireplace and a wildfire raging uncontrolled through a forest. One is contained and serves a purpose: heating a home. The other is uncontrolled and destructive. Both are forms of fire, but the application couldn't be more different.

In the same way, chronic and acute inflammation are two distinct types of inflammatory responses with differing characteristics and impacts on the body. Acute inflammation is like the first kind of fire. It serves a purpose for the greater good of your health. You need inflammation for the healing process to begin. It's a short-term, localized immune response triggered by tissue injury or infection. It's characterized by classic signs such as redness, swelling, heat, pain, and loss of function. Acute inflammation is a protective mechanism to eliminate harmful stimuli and initiate healing. When damaged, tissue releases inflammation signals into the body, which kicks off the healing cascade. You twist your ankle, the tissue swells and gets hot, the swelling goes down, and healing happens. That's the proper application of acute inflammation. Acute inflammation is a natural response by the body to protect and repair damaged tissue. It helps remove harmful substances, pathogens, and damaged cells from the site of injury and promotes the recruitment of immune cells and growth factors to aid in the healing process. While acute inflammation can be painful and uncomfortable, it is a crucial part of the body's natural healing mechanism.

However, this code talks about chronic inflammation, which lasts three months or longer and is destructive to the human body. It's the wildfire burning out of control and wreaking havoc on its surroundings, which are our joints, brain, nerves, muscles, organs, etc. It's a long-lasting, persistent inflammatory response that can happen when acute inflammation fails to resolve or the immune system is continually activated.

Most people with a complex chronic illness have systemic, chronic inflammation and don't realize it. Systemic inflammation, or systemic inflammatory response syndrome (SIRS), refers to inflammation that affects the whole body rather than a specific area or system. It involves the release of inflammatory mediators, such as cytokines, into the bloodstream.

Inflammatory cytokines are signaling molecules released by immune cells to regulate the immune response and inflammation. During systemic inflammation, immune cells produce and release excessive amounts of inflammatory cytokines into the bloodstream. These cytokines, such as interleukin-1 (IL-1), interleukin-6 (IL-6), and tumor necrosis factor-alpha (TNF-alpha), play a pivotal role in triggering and sustaining the systemic inflammatory response.

Various factors, including infections, autoimmune disorders, tissue damage, and exposure to toxins or irritants, can trigger systemic inflammation. The five leading causes of systemic inflammation include:

1. Intestinal Permeability. Better known as leaky gut or leaky gut syndrome, this is a condition in which the lining of

the small intestine become more permeable then normal. In this context, "leaky" refers to the increased passage of molecules (such as toxins, bacteria, and undigested food particles) from the digestive tract into the sterile bloodstream. Leaky gut leads to the release of pro-inflammatory cytokines such as TFN-alpha, Interleukin-6, Interleukin -1 beta, and Interleukin-8. What does this cause? Systemic chronic inflammation and tissue destruction of joints, brain, liver, and kidney as well as other tissues and organs of the body. Leaky gut is also known to be the "gateway" to autoimmunity.

2. Environmental Toxins: We will discuss this code in more detail later in the book, but a few of the multitude of toxins that lead to chronic inflammation and tissue destruction are heavy metals, pesticides, herbicides, plastics, and mycotoxins (mold).

3. Infections: Bacterial or viral infections including dental bacteria like Porphyromnas gingivalis or P. gingivalis and Streptococcus mutans or S. mutans, tick bites containing Borrelia burgdorferi, or fungal infections can induce systemic inflammation in the brain and heart and cause other organ and tissue destruction.

4. Autoimmune Diseases: You may wonder how chronic inflammation progresses to autoimmune diseases Firstly, through the loss of immune tolerance. In autoimmune diseases, the immune system mistakenly identifies the body's own tissues and molecules as foreign invaders and launches an immune response against them. Chronic inflammation can disrupt the body's mechanisms for maintaining immune tolerance, allowing the immune system to attack healthy cells and tissues.

Secondly, through molecular mimicry: some pathogens, environmental factors, and even undigested proteins (gluten, a wheat protein, and casein, a milk protein) can penetrate the gut barrier system, as well as the blood-brain barrier system, and trigger an immune response.

The molecular structure of these antigens may "look like" or "mimic" the molecular structure of the body's cells, tissues or organs, hence the name molecular mimicry, once again tagging the body tissues for destruction. This can lead to a confusion in the immune system, causing it to target both the pathogen and the body's own tissues, leading to an autoimmune response. Conditions like rheumatoid arthritis, systemic lupus erythematosus (SLE), and inflammatory bowel disease (IBD), neurodegeneration leading to dementia, as well as other brain-based disorders can contribute to chronic systemic inflammation, molecular mimicry and autoimmunity.

5. Lifestyle Factors: Lifestyle can significantly contribute to chronic inflammation in the body. Chronic inflammation is associated with a range of health conditions including diabetes, cardiovascular disease, autoimmune diseases, and certain cancers.

Lifestyle can play a pivotal role in promoting chronic inflammation in the following ways:

1. Diet. Pro-inflammatory foods such as processed sugar, fast food, saturated fats and trans fats, refined carbohydrates, gluten and casein can promote inflammation.
2. A sedentary lifestyle is associated with chronic inflammation.

3. Obesity: Excess body fat, especially visceral fat (fat around internal organs), can release pro-inflammatory chemicals called cytokines.
4. Stress. Chronic stress can lead to the release of stress hormones, such as cortisol, which can contribute to inflammation. Excessive cortisol release can also damage the hippocampus which may lead to dementia.
5. Sleep. Poor sleep or chronic sleep deprivation can disrupt the body's natural anti-inflammatory processes, potentially leading to not only increased inflammation, but dementia as well.

Chronic systemic inflammation can devastate the brain, body, and gut. It's associated with an increased risk of various chronic conditions, including cardiovascular disease, type 2 diabetes, autoimmune disorders, neurodegenerative diseases, and gastrointestinal disorders. In the brain, chronic inflammation has been linked to cognitive decline, mood disorders, and an increased risk of neurodegenerative diseases such as Alzheimer's and Parkinson's. Chronic inflammation contributes to tissue damage, organ dysfunction, and an increased risk of chronic diseases in the body. In the gut, it can disrupt the balance of gut microbiota, impair nutrient absorption, and contribute to conditions like inflammatory bowel disease (IBD).

HOW DO YOU KNOW IF YOU HAVE CHRONIC INFLAMMATION?

This code likes to attack the weakest link in the proverbial chain. When a raiding army comes in to attack an enemy, they don't attack the strongest point in the castle. Instead, they find the weakest spot and attack it repeatedly. In the same way, the weakest system in your body is usually the first tissue that submits to the damaging fire of chronic inflammation. The most fragile tissue has the least substrate to fight off its effects.

Because chronic inflammation can manifest itself in so many different ways, it can lead to a variety of symptoms:

- Focus, attention, and concentration issues
- Memory issues such as dementia
- Movement disorders like tremors or early-onset Parkinson's
- Depression or anxiety
- Joint pain
- Thyroid issues
- Digestive disorders
- Poor circulation/cold hands. Cold feet = cold brain.

In addition to symptoms like these, there's another way we can tell if you have chronic inflammation: lab tests that measure the five primary inflammatory markers:

1. A1C: Also known as the hemoglobin A1C or HbA1c test, this simple blood test measures your average blood sugar levels over the past three months. For optimal function, your A1C should be 5.3 or below.
2. C-reactive protein (CRP): The liver makes this protein. The level of CRP increases when there's inflammation in the body. For optimal function your CRP should be below 1.0.

3. Blood sugar: Blood glucose, or blood sugar, is the main sugar in your blood and your body's primary energy source. If blood sugar is high for too long, it can cause an inflammatory response. For optimal function your glucose level should be between 85 and 99.

4. Homocysteine: This is an amino acid: a chemical your body uses to make proteins. Typically, vitamins B12, B6, and folic acid break down homocysteine and change it into other substances your body needs, so there should be very little homocysteine left in your bloodstream. When these levels elevate, inflammation is present, and everyday physiological processes aren't happening. The optimal range for this test is 7.0 or below.

5. A/G ratio: Also known as albumin to globulin ratio, this is a measurement that compares albumin (a protein in the liver) to globulin (a group of proteins that play a role in the immune system) in the blood. It is often included as part of a blood panel or blood test. A/G ratio can provide insights into certain conditions such as liver or kidney disease, infections, inflammation or malabsorption issues. The optimal range for A/G ratio is 1.8 or below.

Have you watched the movie *Titanic*? Do you remember the scene where the ship was sinking after it hit the iceberg, and its crew shot off multiple flare guns, frantically trying to alert nearby vessels that they were in grave danger and needed help? The sailors shot off those flares as alerts, signals that something was wrong, but the bursts didn't tell the other ships what had happened, only that trouble was afoot. These inflammatory markers are a lot like those flares. They tell us there's a fire raging but not where it's located. Your symptoms usually tell me where the inflammation is located such as painful joints, brain fog, anxiety, gut bloating, constipation, etc.

SUB-CODES OF INFLAMMATION

Within this major code exist several "sub-codes" that either point to or create an issue with systemic inflammation. These codes include:

- Gluten sensitivity. This sub-code is relatively straightforward. We use Cyrex Labs array #3x to make a precise diagnosis.
- Leaky gut. Also known as intestinal permeability, the mainstream medical community hardly ever diagnoses this issue. Did you know that research shows 80 to 90% of Americans have a leaky gut? However, many in the medical community roll their eyes at it. Is that because there's no FDA-approved drug currently to treat it? Regardless of Western medicine's attitude towards this condition, knowing about and treating it is vital because it's a major, chronic inflammatory cascade that usually goes systemic. Cyrex Labs array #2 can test for this issue.
- Blood sugar dysregulation. This sub-code means that blood sugar levels are consistently too high. Normal blood sugar levels should be between 85 and 99, and A1C levels should be 5.3 or lower. As discussed in the next chapter, blood sugar dysregulation is one of the most overlooked markers of inflammation. A simple LabCorp blood test can reveal if you have blood sugar dysregulation or not.

- Mold. Research shows that 70% of American households have mold, making this sub-code one of the most overlooked toxins. Using Cyrex Labs array #12 I test my patients for three kinds of mold: Aspergillus, Penicillium and Stachybotrys chartarum (black mold), with black mold the most damaging to the human body.
- Dental pathogens: I test my patients for two dental bacterial infections: Streptococcus mutans (gingivitis) and P. gingivalis (periodontal disease). These bacteria dump into the bloodstream from the mouth and cause systemic inflammation. S. mutans has been linked to movement disorders and P. gingivalis has been to Alzheimer's disease, cardiovascular disease, and rheumatoid arthritis.
- Standard American diet and lifestyle: What you put in your mouth is one of the most significant predictors of your future health. The standard American diet is riddled with processed food, gluten, sugar, and damaging seed oils. Fixing this sub-code is simple: Stop eating processed junk food and start moving your body regularly. There are no lab tests for this one, just buy a mirror and weight scale.

DETECTION AND TREATMENT

The mainstream healthcare field, the "standard of care" system, usually ignores most if not all the of the issues I just shared, with the exception of blood sugar. Still, you don't have to look any further than the scientific research to see that any of these sub-codes could be causing significant systemic inflammation in your body. Regrettably, many healthcare professionals fail to conduct the above comprehensive tests. To crack this unique code, I guide my patients through 10-or-more in-depth metabolic lab tests that reveal the underlying triggers exacerbating their conditions.

Detecting systemic inflammation caused by this code and its sub-codes involves assessing clinical symptoms, conducting laboratory tests (e.g., complete blood count, C-reactive protein, homocysteine, albumin/globulin ratio 1.8 or below, A.I.C. marker), and identifying the underlying infectious agent through specific tests. It also involves a thorough medical history evaluation, physical examination, laboratory tests, and imaging studies, if necessary. Detection may involve assessing body mass index (BMI), waist circumference and performing blood tests to measure markers of inflammation, including C-reactive protein.

PATIENT SUCCESS STORY

About a year ago a patient came to the clinic with several severe symptoms, including chronic pain, neuropathy, and a bent, hunched posture. He came to me after going to several doctors and finding zero relief. We ran several lab tests to find the source of his problem. When the results came back, his codes were screaming "inflammation." A leaky gut and severe gluten sensitivity were the main drivers causing his chronic inflammation. A fire burned inside him, and his standard American diet was pouring gasoline on the flames. Once we knew his codes, we removed gluten from his diet. He improved significantly. He did a brain, body, and gut detox, improving his symptoms even more. He followed my recommended treatment plan for four months, and today, he's walking without a cane. He's no longer hunched, and his neuropathy has significantly decreased. He's happy and has hope for the future. He found a renewed love for traveling, working in his yard, and enjoying his family and friends. Breaking his codes gave him his quality of life back.

The standard healthcare protocol and insurance model doesn't allow healthcare providers to dig this deep or look at inflammatory markers like leaky gut, gluten sensitivity, or mycotoxins (mold). My approach is unique because I leave no stone unturned to determine where your fire is coming from. Whenever a new patient comes in, I see it as rebuilding a house. We're rebuilding that person's body, and when there have been years of damage, it's unrealistic to think that repair will happen immediately. It takes time for the body to lay down enough healthy tissue to heal itself. However, this process is lab-based and scientific. We don't take shots in the dark. Instead, we use precise testing and years of clinical experience to help you break your unique code. See a list of tests and what they do on the next page.

Are you hungry for more insights?
Visit www.thecodebreakeronline.com for an even
deeper dive into the subjects covered in this chapter.

LABCORP - tests fasting glucose levels, A1C, CRP, A/G ratio, homocysteine, vitamin D, and more.

CYREX 2 - tests for intestinal permeability, as well as Lipopolysaccharides (gramma-negative bacteria) that unleashes its destructive powers if it penetrates the gut barrier, leading to chronic inflammation and autoimmunity.

CYREX 3X - tests for gluten sensitivity, wheat germ agglutinin, transglutaminase-2 gut health, transglutaminase-3 skin health, transglutaminase-6 brain and nervous system health and more.

CYREX 4 - gluten cross-reactivity test. It assesses whether there is a cross-reactivity between gluten and other non-gluten proteins. Cross-reactivity means that the immune system may react to other proteins that resemble gluten (molecular mimicry), potentially causing similar reactions.

CYREX5 - A multiple autoimmune reactivity screen and it measures predictive antibodies and self-targeting indicators for acquiring particular autoimmune diseases in the future. It determines potential tissue damage in various organs, including cardiovascular, endocrine, joint, gastrointestinal, and neurological. Antibodies are proteins produced by the immune system in response to the presence of specific antigens, such as pathogens or foreign substances.

CYREX 10 - This panel measures reactivity to 180 food antigens in the cooked, raw, process or modified in one panel.

CREX 11- This panel measures immune reactivity to a wide range of chemicals including mold toxins, detergent chemicals, plastics, flame retardants, dry-cleaning, parabens, heavy metals and more.

CYEX 12 - This test assesses IgG immune reactivity to pathogens that are documented triggers or exacerbators of autoimmunity. This panel tests a variety of pathogens including oral and gastrointestinal pathogens, gastrointestinal parasites, environmental mold, and tick-born pathogens.

CYREX LINX - This panel looks at antibodies to identify your risk and reactivity of triggers for developing neurological disorders. It tests Tau protein antibodies as well as Amyloid-b.

CYREX 22 SIBO - This panel looks at small intestinal bacterial overgrowth.

CHAPTER SIX

CODE #2 BLOOD SUGAR DYSREGULATION

"Being a successful person is not necessarily defined by what you have achieved, but by what you have overcome."

—FANNIE FLAGG

Blood sugar, also known as glucose, is our body's fuel. If the octane level in your car is too high or low, will it run properly? No, absolutely not. Just as your vehicle requires a specific level of octane to perform, the body is also a finely tuned machine that needs a particular glucose range to excel.

When we measure blood sugar through lab work, an at-home blood sugar monitor, or a continuous glucose monitor (CGM), we get something similar to a screenshot of where our blood sugar is at that moment. Another test you're probably familiar with, A1C, is more like a movie. It provides valuable information about long-term blood sugar control over two-to-three months. Both numbers are essential because I've seen patients have excellent blood sugar the day of the blood test. Yet a high A1C indicates that they have blood sugar dysregulation.

Blood sugar matters, because inside every cell in your body you have something akin to tiny nuclear power plants. They're called mitochondria: the structures that make energy to power your cells. Inside the cell, the mitochondria use blood sugar and oxygen to create energy for the body, called Adenosine Triphosphate or ATP. When your blood sugar is dysregulated, you don't have the right fuel for our mitochondria to make energy. Therefore, you may have symptoms such as chronic fatigue or lack of focus, attention, and concentration, numbness, and tingling in your hands and feet.

When blood sugar is consistently over 99, in the range of 100–125, it's called insulin resistance. Blood sugar levels of 126 or higher officially makes you type-2 diabetic. Insulin resistance is a problem because it can trigger not only symptoms as the ones stated above, but it can cause protein aggregation in the brain. This condition happens when the proteins in your brain begin sticking together like Velcro, causing neurons to slow down in their firing rate, thus slowing neurotransmission which may lead to neurodegeneration, neuroinflammation, mental fatigue, and—you guessed it—dementia and Parkinson's disease.

Most people think blood sugar dysregulation only causes neuropathy. However, it can also cause cognitive decline, movement disorders, and balance problems. It's also known to cause heart problems. When your blood sugar is too high, your body takes the excess glucose and turns it into triglycerides, which can cause clogging of the arteries. In the 1980s, a war against good, healthy forms of saturated fat began, and the corporate advertising machine convinced everyone that heart disease came from eating too much fat. However, we now know that was a hoax and that most heart disease and arterial blockages come from eating a diet high in processed carbs and sugar.

For most people, the hamster wheel of blood sugar dysregulation goes like this: Their blood sugar is too high, so they're constantly tired. They drink a 5-Hour Energy to get through the day, and eat a high-carb diet because they're continually crashing from the previous blood sugar spike. They have excess circulating blood sugar which the body converts to triglycerides and is stored in adipose (fat) tissue. This conversion from excessive glucose to triglycerides requires a tremendous amount of energy from the body. That's one reason why our insulin-resistant friends are fatigued, tired or fall asleep after a big meal. On the opposite side of the coin, if you have low blood sugar, you'll be fatigued, irritable, and maybe grumpy before a meal, yet feel refreshed and energetic afterward.

Optimal blood sugar regulation is crucial for maintaining the overall health and functioning of the brain, body, and gut. When blood sugar levels are consistently too high or too low, it can have devastating effects, particularly in insulin resistance and diabetes. There are three main reasons why optimal blood sugar control is essential and how insulin resistance and diabetes can impact the brain, body, and gut:

- Brain Function: The brain relies heavily on a steady supply of glucose, its primary energy source. Amazingly, the human brain weighs just three pounds, about 2% of the body's total weight, but accounts for 20% of glucose and oxygen consumption. Fluctuations in blood sugar levels can disrupt brain function and lead to cognitive impairments, mood disturbances, decreased mental acuity, and problems with focus, attention, and concentration. In conditions like insulin resistance and diabetes, where blood sugar regulation is compromised, the brain may experience chronic exposure to elevated glucose levels, leading to long-term damage. In addition, high blood sugar levels can contribute to the development of conditions like vascular dementia and Alzheimer's disease.

- Body Function: Maintaining optimal blood sugar levels is essential for the proper functioning of various organs and systems within the body. Insulin resistance, the harbinger of type 2 diabetes, occurs when the body's cells become less responsive to the effects of insulin, resulting in elevated blood sugar levels. Prolonged high blood sugar levels can damage blood vessels, nerves, and organs throughout the body. Complications associated with diabetes include cardiovascular disease, kidney disease, nerve damage, eye problems, and impaired wound healing.

- Gut Function: The gut is critical in digestion, nutrient absorption, and overall health. Insulin resistance and diabetes can disrupt gut function and contribute to various gastrointestinal complications. Elevated blood sugar levels can promote the growth of harmful bacteria in the gut, leading to imbalances in the gut microbiome. Furthermore, diabetes can affect the nerves that control digestion, leading to conditions like gastroparesis, which slows down stomach emptying.

Formation of Advanced Glycosylated End Products: When there is too much sugar in the blood (usually due to diabetes), it can stick to proteins, fats, and DNA in the body. This process is called glycation. Over time, these sugar-protein or sugar-fat combinations become advanced glycosylated end products (AGEs). AGEs can form inside the body or come from certain foods we eat, like fried or processed foods.

Impact on the Body: AGEs can cause problems in our cells. They can change the structure of proteins, making them work differently or not at all. For example, they can affect the collagen in blood vessels, making them less flexible and causing stiffness. AGEs can also interact with specific receptors in our cells, leading to inflammation, oxidative stress, and the release of harmful substances.

Consequences and Complications: The buildup of AGEs in the body has been linked to complications associated with diabetes. They can contribute to kidney problems, eye damage, nerve damage, and heart disease. AGEs cause inflammation, oxidative stress, and damage to blood vessels, which are all factors in these complications. Additionally, they can lead to the production of substances that cause tissue scarring and impaired organ function.

DETECTION AND TREATMENT

Ideally, we want our blood sugar to stay steady without significant spikes and dips. You may already know if your blood sugar is too high or low, but if you've never had your blood sugar or A1C levels tested, here are a few questions to ask yourself:

1. Do you often fall asleep after big meals, especially those high in carbohydrates? This can indicate a level of insulin resistance.
2. Do you often have headaches, feel sluggish, or get "hangry" if you don't eat for long periods? This can indicate hypoglycemia, aka low blood sugar.
3. Do you need help with focus, attention, and concentration?
4. Are you consistently physically fatigued?
5. Are your triglycerides too high or low?
6. Do you have neuropathy, numbness, and tingling in your hands or feet?
7. Are you overweight or underweight?
8. Do you have a high BMI of over 25?

9. Do you consistently eat an unhealthy diet of processed foods, sugar, and inflammatory oils such as soybean oil, corn oil, or sunflower oil?

10. Do you have intense, almost unbearable cravings for sugar and carbs?

All of the symptoms listed above can indicate blood sugar dysregulation. When patients ask me, "Dr. Barlow, what causes blood sugar issues?" many don't like the answer because blood sugar dysregulation is usually a self-inflicted problem. This discourages a lot of people. They think, "Oh no, I did this to myself. I caused this problem." While that may be true, I see it through the lens of hope because that means you can do something about your current situation! If you caused it, you can reverse it.

This code is a disease accumulating over years of poor dietary and lifestyle choices. So how do we reverse it? Do the opposite of what got you there in the first place. As Will Rogers said, "If you find yourself in a hole, stop digging." Cut out sweet tea, soda, and processed junk food. Stop eating inflammatory seed oils (sunflower, canola, corn), fried food, and fast food. Turn away from the standard American diet. Instead, eat real, whole foods, move your body consistently, and drink enough water—at least a half a gallon per day. Cutting out sugar, gluten, and processed food and adding in a 30-minute daily walk will change your life. Exercise burns off glucose, and one of the simplest and most enjoyable forms of exercise, walking, is very effective at helping the body process glucose.

Walking also releases a neurotransmitter called dopamine, which is associated with pleasure, reward, and motivation. Engaging in physical activity like walking stimulates the release of dopamine in the brain leading to a sense of pleasure and well-being. Walking can also activate serotonin, which is another neurotransmitter that plays a crucial role in mood regulation, happiness, and relaxation. Physical activity, including walking, has been shown to stimulate the release of serotonin in the brain. Walking outdoors in natural environments can have an even greater impact on serotonin levels. Being in nature and receiving sunlight exposure can further boost serotonin production and contribute to a positive and relaxed state of mind.

These principles are simple and effective, but they're not always easy. Many patients are reluctant to make lifestyle changes. They'd rather pop a pill and keep drinking sweet tea. Those people rarely break their codes and reclaim their life. The patients with the most success commit to doing whatever it takes to regain their health. They realize the only thing they're losing is a liability, and they make the changes necessary to become a code breaker. You have one life to live, so live it to the max!

If you want to slow down, reverse, or prevent any of the seven codes to complex chronic illness, eating the opposite of the standard American diet and moving your body for 30 minutes per day, five days per week, will help you do that. If you can't walk for 30 minutes, start with five minutes per day. Then build up to 10 minutes, then 20. Soon, you'll be walking for 30 minutes like a champ.

PATIENT SUCCESS STORIES

One middle-aged woman came in with chronic knee pain. She was overweight and followed the standard American diet. She had widespread systemic inflammation, and we learned she had a gluten intolerance through Cyrex lab testing. I suggested she change her diet, eliminating gluten, processed food, and sugar, and do the 10-week brain, body, and gut detox. These changes helped her get the inflammation under control and stabilized her blood sugar. To my amazement, she became virtually pain-free in under 12 weeks.

A different patient came in with complaints of severe neuropathy. The typical medical prescription for such a problem is Gabapentin, which appears to work by altering electrical activity in the brain and influencing the activity of chemicals called neurotransmitters, which send messages between nerve cells. Side effects of the drug may include brain fog, slight confusion, and memory impairment: ouch! The drug may help with the pain for a while, but it's a band-aid that doesn't fix the root cause of the blood sugar problem or regenerate the nerve damage. I suggested this patient get off the standard American diet and do the 10-week detox. She also did weekly therapy in the clinic. She lost weight, her blood sugar stabilized, and the neuropathy disappeared. We removed the triggers and allowed the body to heal itself.

This patient's story shows that understanding and managing blood sugar levels is paramount for optimal health and well-being. Like the precise octane level needed for a car to run smoothly, the body requires a specific glucose range to function at its best. Blood sugar dysregulation can have far-reaching consequences, impacting our energy levels, focus, and cognitive abilities such as depression and anxiety. When blood sugar is consistently too high, it can lead to insulin resistance and protein aggregation, causing chronic health issues and heart problems.

On the other hand, low blood sugar can result in persistent fatigue and exhaustion. Recognizing the importance of balanced blood sugar levels is crucial in breaking free from the hamster wheel of energy fluctuations and paving the way toward a more vibrant and thriving life. By cracking this code and achieving a state of insulin sensitivity and balanced blood sugar, we can fuel our bodies optimally and support the intricate power plants within our cells, the mitochondria, to produce the energy needed for a healthier, more fulfilling life.

Are you hungry for more insights?
Visit www.thecodebreakeronline.com for an even
deeper dive into the subjects covered in this chapter.

CHAPTER SEVEN

CODE #3 MALABSORPTION SYNDROME

"You don't have to be great to start, but you have to start to be great."

—ZIG ZIGLAR

Have you ever heard the saying, "It's not how much you earn; it's how much you keep?" You can earn $1,000,000 annually, but your bank account will look abysmal if you spend $1,000,0001. Well, digestion is similar. It's not always about how much you eat or what you eat; it's about how much your body can absorb and utilize.

This code, malabsorption, refers to the impaired absorption of nutrients from the gastrointestinal tract into the bloodstream. Having this code leads to an inability to draw nutrition from food, depriving the body of the raw materials needed to heal. To create healthy new cells, we must have the substrate and raw materials for the body to heal itself. Malabsorption can devastate the human brain, body, and gut because it deprives the body of essential nutrients, minerals, amino acids, carbohydrates, and healthy fats for optimal functioning.

Vitamin A plays a crucial role in maintaining overall health and well-being. Here are some key reasons why it is important:

1. Vision: Vitamin A is essential for good vision, particularly in low-light conditions. It helps form a pigment called rhodopsin in the eyes, which enables us to see in dim light and improves night vision.

2. Immune function: Vitamin A supports a healthy immune system by promoting the production and function of white blood cells, which defend the body against infections and diseases. It also helps maintain the integrity of the skin and mucous membranes, acting as a barrier against pathogens.
3. Growth and development: For children, vitamin A is vital for normal growth and development. It contributes to the formation and maintenance of healthy teeth, bones, and soft tissues.
4. Reproduction and fetal development: Vitamin A is important for reproductive health in both males and females. It plays a role in sperm production and the development of the placenta during pregnancy.
5. Cell differentiation: Vitamin A is involved in the process of cell differentiation, where immature cells mature into specialized cells with specific functions. This process is crucial for normal organ development and maintenance.
6. Antioxidant properties: As an antioxidant, vitamin A helps protect cells from damage caused by harmful molecules called free radicals. This can help prevent chronic diseases and reduce the risk of certain cancers.

To ensure sufficient vitamin A intake, it is recommended to consume a balanced diet that includes foods rich in this essential nutrient, such as liver, fish, dairy products, eggs, carrots, sweet potatoes, spinach, and other leafy greens.

B vitamins are a group of essential nutrients that play a crucial role in maintaining overall health. They include thiamine (B1), riboflavin (B2), niacin (B3), pantothenic acid (B5), pyridoxine

(B6), biotin (B7), folate (B9), and cobalamin (B12). Here's why they are important:

1. Energy production: B vitamins are involved in converting the food we eat into energy. They help in the metabolism of carbohydrates, proteins, and fats, providing the body with the energy it needs to function properly.
2. Red blood cell formation: Certain B vitamins, such as folate and cobalamin, are necessary for the production of healthy red blood cells. They play a crucial role in preventing anemia and ensuring optimal oxygen transport throughout the body.
3. Nervous system function: B vitamins are essential for maintaining a healthy nervous system. They are involved in the production of neurotransmitters, which facilitate communication between nerve cells. This supports proper brain function and can contribute to mood regulation.
4. DNA synthesis and cell division: B vitamins, particularly folate and cobalamin, are vital for DNA synthesis and cell division. They are crucial during periods of rapid growth and development, such as pregnancy and infancy.
5. Heart health: Certain B vitamins, like riboflavin, niacin, and B6, are important for cardiovascular health. They help in maintaining normal cholesterol levels, supporting healthy blood vessels, and reducing the risk of heart diseases.
6. Skin, hair, and nail health: B vitamins are involved in maintaining the health of the skin, hair, and nails. They promote cell growth and repair, ensuring healthy tissues and preventing conditions like dermatitis and hair loss.

7. Mood regulation: B vitamins, particularly thiamine, niacin, and B6, are essential for the production of neurotransmitters involved in mood regulation. Adequate levels of these vitamins can contribute to a balanced mood and help prevent conditions like depression and anxiety.

It is important to consume a balanced diet that includes foods rich in B vitamins or consider supplementation if necessary, especially for individuals with certain dietary restrictions or conditions that may affect absorption.

Vitamin D is essential for overall health due to the following reasons:

1. Bone health: Vitamin D plays a crucial role in calcium absorption and bone mineralization. It helps regulate the levels of calcium and phosphate in the body, which are necessary for maintaining strong and healthy bones. Sufficient vitamin D levels help prevent conditions like rickets in children and osteoporosis in adults.

2. Immune function: Vitamin D helps regulate the immune system, enabling it to function optimally. It plays a role in the production and regulation of immune cells, thereby enhancing the body's ability to fight off infections and diseases.

3. Muscle strength: Adequate vitamin D levels are associated with improved muscle strength and function. It helps maintain muscle mass and supports muscle performance, reducing the risk of falls and fractures, especially in older individuals.

4. Mental health: Some studies have suggested a link between vitamin D deficiency and an increased risk of mental health disorders such as depression, anxiety, and seasonal affective disorder (SAD). Adequate vitamin D levels may contribute to overall mental well-being.

5. Heart health: Vitamin D may have a protective effect on cardiovascular health. It has been associated with a lower risk of developing heart disease, hypertension, and other cardiovascular conditions.

6. Cancer prevention: There is emerging evidence that suggests vitamin D may play a role in reducing the risk of certain cancers, including colorectal, breast, and prostate cancers. However, more research is needed to fully understand this relationship.

The primary source of vitamin D is sunlight, as the skin produces it when exposed to UVB rays. However, it can also be obtained through certain foods, such as fatty fish, and supplements. It is essential to maintain adequate vitamin D levels through a combination of proper sun exposure, diet, and supplementation if necessary, especially in individuals who have limited sun exposure or are at higher risk of deficiency.

There are four leading causes of malabsorption:

1. Celiac Disease: an autoimmune disorder triggered by ingesting gluten, a protein found in wheat, barley, and rye. When individuals with celiac disease consume gluten, their immune system responds by damaging the lining of the small intestine, leading to malabsorption. Over time, this can result in deficiencies of vital nutrients such as iron, calcium, and vitamins. Detecting celiac disease

and associated malabsorption can be done through blood tests that measure levels of specific antibodies, such as anti-tissue transglutaminase (tTG) antibodies. My favorite test is Cyrex array 3x.

2. Non-celiac gluten sensitivity (NCGS): a condition in which individuals experience symptoms similar to those of celiac disease, such as gastrointestinal discomfort and fatigue, but without the autoimmune response and damage to the small intestine. There is evidence to suggest that NCGS may be associated with malabsorption. Don't guess: test, using Cyrex array 3x.

3. Leaky Gut: increased intestinal permeability, where the lining of the small intestine becomes more porous, allowing substances such as toxins, bacteria, and undigested food particles to pass through into the bloodstream. A quick Google search reveals 80 to 90% of Americans have a leaky gut, yet this condition isn't universally recognized in mainstream medicine. Shocker right? Increased permeability of the intestinal lining could potentially lead to the inefficient absorption of nutrients, as a damaged or compromised barrier might allow large molecules to enter the bloodstream, triggering an immune response, inflammation and immune antibody production. A quick reminder that leaky gut is the gateway to autoimmunity. How do we test for this intestinal permeability? Cyrex array #2.

4. Small Intestinal Bacterial Overgrowth (SIBO): This is a condition where there is an excessive growth of bacteria in the small intestine. This overgrowth can disrupt the normal digestion and absorption of nutrients, potentially leading to malabsorption. The overgrowth of bacteria

in the small intestine can compete with the host for nutrients. These bacteria can consume nutrients before they have a chance to be absorbed by the body, leading to malabsorption of essential vitamins, mineral, proteins, fats, and carbohydrates. We can test for the presence of SIBO using Cyrex Labs array #22.

So what causes this code? Like the other codes, several things can trigger its existence. Brain trauma, gluten sensitivity, processed food, a diet high in sugar and carbohydrates, nonsteroidal anti-inflammatory drugs (NSAIDs) like aspirin or ibuprofen, long term use of antibiotics, or not producing enough hydrochloric acid can all lead to malabsorption syndrome over time. Being over age 60 means you're probably not producing enough hydrochloric acid, known as hypochlorhydria.

Hypochlorhydria refers to low stomach acid production, which can occur due to various factors such as aging, certain medications, chronic stress, or underlying health conditions. The link between hypochlorhydria and malabsorption is particularly strong when it comes to certain nutrients like B vitamins.

Low stomach acid can impair the breakdown and digestion of food, especially proteins. This can lead to poor absorption of essential nutrients, including B vitamins, which require sufficient stomach acid for their release from food and subsequent binding with proteins for absorption. In the absence of adequate stomach acid, the absorption of B vitamins, particularly vitamin B12, can be compromised.

Vitamin B12 deficiency is commonly associated with hypochlorhydria and malabsorption issues, because it is predominantly found in animal-derived foods and requires stomach acid and an intrinsic factor (a protein produced in the stomach) for absorption. When there is insufficient stomach acid, the intrinsic factor may not be released adequately, leading to reduced vitamin B12 absorption and potential deficiency.

It is worth noting that other nutrients, such as iron, calcium, and zinc, may also be affected by hypochlorhydria and subsequent malabsorption. These nutrients require an acidic environment for optimal absorption, and low stomach acid levels can hinder their bioavailability.

DETECTION AND TREATMENT

Common symptoms of malabsorption may include chronic diarrhea, weight loss, fatigue, bloating, abdominal pain, nutrient deficiencies, and neurological symptoms like cognitive impairment and mood disturbances.

A total protein and albumin/globulin (A/G) ratio test is one way to know if you have malabsorption syndrome. This test measures the total amount of protein in your blood. There are two major types of protein in the blood: albumin, which helps keep blood from leaking out of blood vessels. It also helps move hormones, medicines, vitamins, and other essential substances throughout the body. Albumin is made in the liver. Then there are globulins, which help fight infection and move nutrients throughout the body. The liver makes some globulins. The immune system makes others. The test also compares the amount of albumin in your blood to the amount of globulin. The comparison is called the albumin/globulin (A/G) ratio and an A/G of 1.8 or below is optimal.

PATIENT SUCCESS STORY

A female in her forties came into my clinic. She was thin, weighing around 101 pounds. You'd look at her on the street and think, "She looks trim and fit; there's no way she's unhealthy." But the reality was that she was struggling with awful gastro-intestinal issues and had severe malabsorption. We ran several tests only to discover that she had NCGS and was ravaged by gluten. She changed her diet and did the 10-week detox plan. A few months later, her mother came into the clinic and said, "Thank you so much for what you did for my daughter. She's so excited because she can gain a little weight now." Malabsorption issues can result in various signs and symptoms, which can vary depending on the specific nutrients that are not being absorbed properly, so if you are suffering with symptoms of diarrhea, steatorrhea (foul-smelling, greasy stools), abdominal bloating, flatulence, mood swings, depression or anxiety, now would be a great time to test yourself for malabsorption syndrome.

How did we break the code?

Lab panels: LabCorp for A/G ratio, Cyrex #2, #3x, #4, #10 and #22.

Are you hungry for more insights?
Visit www.thecodebreakeronline.com for an even
deeper dive into the subjects covered in this chapter.

CHAPTER EIGHT

CODE #4 TOXIC LOAD

"Life has no limitations, except the ones you make."

—Les Brown

According to the CDC website, we're exposed to over 700,000 chemicals and toxins daily. Wow, that's a lot. From perfumes to cleaning products, cosmetics to plastic water bottles, much of your everyday life includes exposure to chemicals that aren't good for your health. So unsurprisingly, code number four is "toxic load," which may include but is not limited to parasites, tick bites, Lyme, bacteria, viruses, heavy metals, pesticides, and herbicides. Suppose you're currently dealing with a complex chronic illness. What healthcare professional have you seen who has mentioned, let alone recommended testing for just one of the above-named toxins? My guess is none. I'm a pretty good guesser.

Our environment is filled with toxins that can significantly impact our brain, body, and gut function. These environmental toxins, such as black mold (Stachybotrys chartarum), plastics, and heavy metals, can sneak into your life without realizing it. Current research shows that 70% of American households have mold in them. Many everyday household items like paint, cleaning products, plastics, herbicides, and pesticides are also highly toxic to our health. I know that 700,000 exposures per day are alarming, so let me put your mind at ease. This chapter aims to help you identify the major toxins in your life and eliminate them so your body can heal. The healthier you get, the better you can handle the other minor exposures in your daily doings.

SIGNIFICANT CONTRIBUTORS TO TOXIC OVERLOAD

There are several sources of toxic exposure you may encounter daily. The key to breaking this code is identifying and removing the toxic items from your life. Here are five of the top sources of toxic load:

1. Mold: One of the most overlooked contributors to toxic load is mold. With research showing 70% of households have mold, statistically, either you have it or your neighbor has it. Think about that for a minute. Why aren't more doctors paying attention to this?

2. Plastics: These are everywhere: food packaging, Tupperware, plastic food storage bags, consumer goods packaging, and more. Using plastic products leads to ingesting and inhaling large amounts of microplastic particles and hundreds of toxic substances with known or suspected carcinogenic, developmental, or endocrine-disrupting impacts.

3. Herbicides and Pesticides: You can be exposed to herbicides and pesticides in various places, including at home, school, or work. They can enter your body by eating, drinking, breathing, and skin contact. Commonly used weed killers like Round-Up are a significant source of toxic exposure to millions of Americans.

4. Dental Amalgam: Did you know the silver-colored fillings in your mouth probably contain mercury, one of

the most potent neurotoxins on earth? Dental amalgam is a mixture of metals consisting of liquid (elemental) mercury and a powdered alloy composed of silver, tin, and copper.

5. Parasites: This category includes worms, protozoa, infections from tick bites like Lyme disease, and more. Common causes of parasitic infections include spending time in areas with known parasites, ingesting contaminated water, foods, soil, blood, or feces (poop), and not washing your hands before eating or drinking.

DETECTION AND TREATMENT

Here are four primary examples of environmental toxins and their effects, along with detection methods:

1. Mold: Black mold, also known as Stachybotrys chartarum, is a toxic mold commonly found in damp and water-damaged environments. When exposed to black mold spores, you may inhale or come into contact with mycotoxins produced by the mold. Prolonged exposure to black mold can lead to respiratory problems, allergic reactions, and other health issues. Detecting black mold involves visual inspection to identify signs of mold growth, such as discoloration or a musty odor. Air quality testing can be conducted to assess mold spore levels in the indoor environment. Warning symptoms of mold exposure include brain fog, memory loss, dizziness, ear infection, headaches and migraines, joint pain, numbness, and tingling in extremities. Additionally, testing

of affected surfaces or materials for mold presence and mycotoxin analysis may be performed in specialized laboratories. We test for this toxin using Cyrex array #12.

2. Plastics: They contain various chemicals, including bisphenol A (BPA) and phthalates, which can leach into food, beverages, and the environment. These chemicals are endocrine-disrupting compounds and can interfere with hormone regulation in the body. Prolonged exposure to plastics and their associated chemicals has adverse effects on reproductive health, hormonal imbalances, and an increased risk of certain diseases. We test for this toxin using Cyrex array #11. Detecting the presence of plastics and associated chemicals in the environment can be challenging. However, some steps to reduce exposure include using BPA-free plastics, avoiding microwaving food in plastic containers, and opting for glass or stainless steel containers for food and drink storage. Suppose your results come back positive for sensitivity to plastic. In that case, you must stop drinking from plastic bottles, using plastic food storage containers, etc. Once your exposure to plastic is limited, we detox your body through antioxidants like glutathione and ensure your liver is functioning correctly. A healthy liver helps you detox from all of these toxins.

3. Heavy Metals: Lead, mercury, cadmium, and arsenic, can be found naturally in the environment or introduced through industrial activities. These metals can accumulate in the body over time and cause toxic effects. Heavy metal exposure has been linked to various health problems, including neurological disorders, impaired

cognitive function, kidney damage, and cardiovascular issues. Detecting heavy metal exposure involves blood, urine, or hair analysis to measure metal levels in the body. Occupational or environmental assessments can also be conducted to identify potential sources of heavy metal exposure. We test for this sub-code using Cyrex array #11.

4. Chemicals: herbicides, pesticides, paint, cleaning products, etc. It's important to note that the impacts of environmental toxins can vary depending on your level of exposure, susceptibility, and overall health. Minimizing exposure to toxins is critical to reducing associated health risks. Implementing preventive measures, such as maintaining a clean and well-ventilated living environment, avoiding direct contact with toxic substances, using protective equipment when necessary, and following proper safety guidelines, can mitigate the harmful effects of environmental toxins.

THE PROCESS OF LIVER DETOXIFICATION

Phase 1: Enzymes called cytochrome P450s are primarily involved. During this phase, enzymes in the liver break down toxins into smaller, less harmful substances. This transformation can create intermediate metabolites that may be more reactive and potentially harmful if not further processed.

Phase 2: Detoxification is the second step, which involves a conjugation reaction (conjugation is a process in which a molecule—an intermediate metabolite—is combined with another molecule to form a larger complex where these intermediate byproducts from Phase 1 are further converted into water-soluble compounds that are readily excreted from the body. This process involves the addition of various molecules, such as amino acids, sulfur, methyl groups, glutathione, glucuronic acid, or acetyl groups, to make the substances less harmful and more quickly eliminated.

In simple terms, Phase 1 detoxification starts breaking down toxins, but it can produce potentially harmful byproducts. Phase 2 detoxification helps convert these byproducts into safer forms that are easily eliminated through urine or stools.

Both phases work together to effectively remove toxins from the body and support overall liver health. It's important to note that a balanced and healthy diet, adequate hydration, and lifestyle choices can play a significant role in supporting these detoxification processes.

Foods that optimize Phase 1 and Phase 2 liver detoxification include brassica vegetables such as cauliflower, cabbage, kale, bok choy, broccoli, Brussels sprouts, turnips, onions, and garlic, as well as citrus fruits, lemon water, ginger drinks, turmeric tea, and green tea.

Foods to avoid during your 10-week detox program to optimize liver function include refined sugars, refined grains, meats, eggs, and dairy.

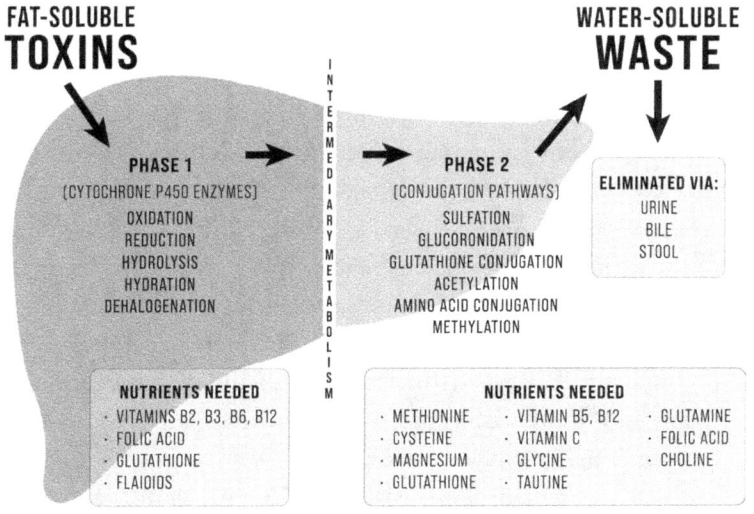

FAT-SOLUBLE
TOXINS

WATER-SOLUBLE
WASTE

INTERMEDIARY METABOLISM

PHASE 1
(CYTOCHRONE P450 ENZYMES)
OXIDATION
REDUCTION
HYDROLYSIS
HYDRATION
DEHALOGENATION

PHASE 2
(CONJUGATION PATHWAYS)
SULFATION
GLUCORONIDATION
GLUTATHIONE CONJUGATION
ACETYLATION
AMINO ACID CONJUGATION
METHYLATION

ELIMINATED VIA:
URINE
BILE
STOOL

NUTRIENTS NEEDED
- VITAMINS B2, B3, B6, B12
- FOLIC ACID
- GLUTATHIONE
- FLAIOIDS

NUTRIENTS NEEDED
- METHIONINE
- CYSTEINE
- MAGNESIUM
- GLUTATHIONE
- VITAMIN B5, B12
- VITAMIN C
- GLYCINE
- TAUTINE
- GLUTAMINE
- FOLIC ACID
- CHOLINE

PATIENT SUCCESS STORIES

My friend spent most of his life in Arizona, but as an adult, he and his family moved to Virginia. Two years after moving to Virginia, he and his family's health took a turn for the worse. It seemed like his entire family started having strange symptoms out of nowhere. It got so bad that he told me, "When I woke up each morning, my first thought was, 'Do I go to the office or the emergency room?'" Their health problem remained unsolved until the day his wife came across a TV show called "Mystery Diagnosis." My friend watched the show in amazement. His family had all the symptoms of the people on the TV show. What was the mystery diagnosis, you might ask? Stachybotrys chartarum, aka black mold. Yet not one doctor had even mentioned running a test for mold. My friend had to move out of his home for a while to remove the mold, and he and his family went through a mold detox program. Today, life is great. Identify the trigger, remove the trigger, detox, and let the body heal.

Another memorable patient story was of a woman who came to my clinic as a "professional patient" and "chronic complainer." Her previous doctors had repeatedly told her, "There's nothing wrong with you. You're imagining things." Still, she knew something wasn't right with her health. She suffered from extreme anxiety, depression, and insomnia and struggled to find hope for the future, but she still wanted to get better and reclaim her joy and life. I listened to her story, completed a neurological exam, and ran ten lab tests. We left no stone unturned to break her previously unsolved codes. The results showed that she had significant black mold exposure, leaky gut, gluten and casein sensitivity, and sensitivity to plastics. She removed the mold from her home, did an intensive mold detox, as well as the brain-body-gut 10 week detox, minimized her exposure to plastics, and eliminated both gluten and casein from her diet. She was committed to doing whatever it took to fix her problem. As a result, her anxiety, depression, and insomnia disappeared.

These accounts are just two of the many success stories. These toxic exposures are everywhere, so it's just a shot in the dark unless you do specific testing. Don't guess: test! You need to figure out what's causing the problem. We go into these tests with zero bias or preconceived ideas. We do the lab work and let the results tell the story. These tests quantify and objectify reality. And with every patient, I do a complete neurological exam to determine systems that are damaged and need help being turned back on. Pair this approach with metabolically testing and removing the triggers, focusing on optimal health—not a band-aid—and you have exceptional healthcare that breaks tough codes.

Are you hungry for more insights?
Visit www.thecodebreakeronline.com for an even
deeper dive into the subjects covered in this chapter.

CHAPTER NINE

CODE #5 VASCULAR HEALTH

"The two most important days in your life are the day you are born and the day you find out why."

—MARK TWAIN

Think of your vascular system as the interstate highway inside your body, except this interstate doesn't transport cars, trucks, and RVs; it's the freeway for your blood, and everything transported in it. The U.S. interstate highway system is approximately 48,191miles in total length. In comparison, our circulatory system has thousands of miles of blood vessels. Estimates vary, but it's generally believed to be around 60,000 to 100,000 miles of blood vessels, when all the arteries, veins, and capillaries are taken into account. These vessels transport blood throughout the body, supplying oxygen, nutrients, glucose, white blood cells, and amino acids, which are protein building blocks that assist in tissue repair, enzyme creation, and metabolism. The blood also supplies a nerve growth component called brain-derived neurotrophic factors (BDNF), which play a crucial role in the growth, maintenance, and survival of neurons. As I tell my patients quite often, "All the healing is in your blood." Your blood contains everything your body needs to heal. We will talk more about this later, but for now, let's talk about blood pressure.

BLOOD PRESSURE:

Optimal blood pressure typically refers to a blood pressure reading within a specific healthy range. The standard guidelines for optimal range are: 1) Systolic pressure (the top number) at 120 mm Hg 2) Diastolic pressure (the bottom number) at 80 mm Hg. This reading is often expressed "120/80 mm Hg" and is considered normal or optimal. However, it's important to note that individual blood pressure can vary based on factors such as age, underlying health conditions, and risk factors. Optimal blood pressure is important because it helps to ensure proper functioning of your cardiovascular system, brain health, gastro-intestinal health, kidney function, eye health, and overall health.

Here's how blood pressure relates to other areas of your health:

1. Heart health: Maintaining optimal blood pressure reduces the strain on your heart. High blood pressure (hypertension) forces the heart to work harder to pump blood, which can lead to heart disease and other cardio-vascular problems.
2. Stroke prevention: Optimal blood pressure is a must for optimal brain function. High blood pressure is a major risk factor for stroke. When blood pressure is too high, it can damage blood vessels in the brain, increasing the risk of stroke. There is also a link between hypertension and vascular dementia.
3. Gastrointestinal health: Studies show that hypertension is associated with increased sympathetic nerve activity (the "fight or flight" branch of the autonomic nervous system).

This increases gut permeability, also known as leaky gut syndrome.

4. Kidney function: The kidneys play a crucial role in regulating blood pressure. High blood pressure, as well as high glucose level, can damage the kidneys over time, leading to kidney disease and kidney failure.

5. Eye health: Hypertension can cause damage to blood vessels in your eyes, potentially leading to vision problems or even blindness.

6. Overall health: High blood pressure is linked to various health issues including risk of heart attack, dementia, and other chronic conditions.

7. Quality of life: Optimal blood pressure promotes overall well-being and helps you feel your best, as it ensures that your organs and tissues receive adequate oxygen, glucose, and nutrients.

To maintain optimal blood pressure, it's essential to adopt a healthy lifestyle, which includes a balanced diet, regular exercise, and stress management: basically, what this entire book is about.

Now let's talk about the brain, spinal cord and gastrointestinal (GI) tract in their relationship to optimal blood flow. Your brain has 86 billion (with a B) nerve cells (neurons). Your spinal cord has 69 million neurons and your gut has 500 million neurons. The gut is often referred to as the "second brain" because of its complex and extensive neuronal network, known as the enteric nervous system (ENS), which is found in the lining of the gastrointestinal tract. Another interesting fact, unbeknownst to most people, is that 70% of your immune system is inside your gut. It's called the gut-associated lymphoid tissue or GALT. Ok, here's where the numbers get even crazier. Ready?

Each neuron in the brain, spinal cord, and GI tract has on average 7,000 synaptic connections (a specialized junction that allows neurons to communicate with each other). This means, on average one neuron communicates with 7,000 other neurons. Could you imagine communicating with 7,000 people at one time? Probably not. The human brain has approximately 600 trillion (with a T) synapses, (86 billion neurons times 7,000 synapses per neuron); the spinal cord has approximately 483 billion (with a B) synapses, and the gastrointestinal tract 3.5 trillion synapses (with a T). Each neuron, along with its 7,000 synapses, relies on a continuous and stable supply of oxygen, glucose, and nutrients to function optimally. This essential supply is delivered to the neurons and synapses located in the brain, spinal cord and gastrointestinal tract through a vital transport system: the bloodstream.

Poor vascular health also refers to compromised blood vessel function, which can significantly negatively impact the brain, body, and gut. This code can lead to reduced blood flow and oxygen supply to the brain, resulting in cognitive impairments, memory problems, and an increased risk of stroke. When blood vessels become narrow, blocked, or damaged, they can disrupt the delivery of essential nutrients, glucose, and oxygen to brain cells, leading to brain tissue damage and neurological deficits. Conditions like cerebral small vessel disease and atherosclerosis can contribute to poor vascular health in the brain.

In the body, poor vascular health affects various organs and systems. When blood vessels become narrowed or damaged, they can impair blood flow to vital organs such as the heart, kidneys, and limbs. Reduced blood supply to these organs can lead to conditions like coronary artery disease, peripheral artery disease, and chronic kidney disease.

In the gut, the gastrointestinal tract is richly supplied with blood vessels that support proper digestion, absorption, and overall gut function. Poor vascular health in the gut can lead to conditions like mesenteric ischemia, where the blood supply to the intestines is compromised. Reduced blood flow can cause abdominal pain, intestinal damage, and impaired nutrient absorption.

When patients enter my clinic, I test their blood pressure to see if they have optimal blood flow. During the neurological exam, I also take the temperature of their hands and feet, and I measure the saturated oxygen carried in the red blood cells with a pulse oximeter. I want to know if oxygen and blood flow are reaching their body's distal extremities (fingers and toes). These tests matter because if you have cold hands and cold feet, along with a low pulse oximeter score, you may have a "cold brain," depriving the brain of blood and oxygen. Insufficient blood flow and oxygen at the distal extremities may equate to insufficient blood and oxygen to the brain.

So, what is the root cause of this often overlooked code? There are several, but I will focus on the three primary sources I often see in my patients:

1. Thyroid: The thyroid gland plays a significant role in regulating the cardiovascular system. It produces and releases thyroid hormones, primarily triiodothyronine (T3) and thyroxine (T4), which have a direct impact on cardiovascular function. Here are several ways in which the thyroid gland influences the cardiovascular system:

> a. Heart Rate and Rhythm: Thyroid hormones have a stimulatory effect on the heart, increasing heart rate and enhancing the force of contraction.

They also help regulate the electrical impulses that control the heart's rhythm. Excessive thyroid hormone levels (hyperthyroidism) can lead to tachycardia (rapid heart rate) and irregular heart rhythms, such as atrial fibrillation.

b. Blood Pressure: Thyroid hormones influence blood pressure regulation. Increased levels of thyroid hormones can cause dilation of blood vessels, leading to decreased peripheral resistance and lower blood pressure. On the other hand, low thyroid hormone levels (hypothyroidism) can result in increased peripheral resistance and higher blood pressure.

c. Cardiac Output: Thyroid hormones have a direct effect on cardiac output, which is the amount of blood pumped by the heart per minute. They increase the heart's contractility and enhance the overall efficiency of the heart's pumping action. As a result, hyperthyroidism can lead to an increased cardiac output, while hypothyroidism can decrease it.

d. Lipid Profile: Thyroid hormones influence lipid metabolism, including the synthesis, breakdown, and clearance of cholesterol and triglycerides. Hyperthyroidism often leads to elevated levels of circulating lipids, including cholesterol. This can increase the risk of atherosclerosis and cardiovascular disease. Hypothyroidism, on the other hand, can cause elevated levels of total cholesterol and LDL cholesterol.

e. Vasodilation and Vasoconstriction: Thyroid hormones affect the tone of blood vessels, regulating their constriction and dilation. They promote the production of nitric oxide, a potent vasodilator that helps relax blood vessel walls. Additionally, thyroid hormones can modulate the sensitivity of blood vessels to other vasoconstrictors and vasodilators, affecting overall vascular tone and blood flow.

f. Coagulation and Fibrinolysis: Thyroid hormones influence the coagulation and fibrinolysis processes, which are responsible for blood clotting and dissolution of blood clots, respectively. Hyperthyroidism can lead to a hypercoagulable state, increasing the risk of thrombosis. Hypothyroidism, on the other hand, can cause impaired fibrinolysis, making it more difficult to dissolve blood clots.

Overall, the thyroid gland exerts significant control over the cardiovascular system through the production and release of thyroid hormones. Imbalances in thyroid hormone levels can disrupt the normal functioning of the heart, blood vessels, and blood coagulation processes, potentially leading to cardiovascular complications. Therefore, proper thyroid function is essential for maintaining a healthy cardiovascular system.

2. Brain Trauma: Head trauma, particularly severe traumatic brain injury (TBI), can have various effects on the cardiovascular system. Here are some ways head trauma can impact cardiovascular health:

a. Autonomic dysfunction: Head trauma can disrupt the functioning of the autonomic nervous system, which controls involuntary bodily functions, including heart rate and blood pressure regulation. This dysfunction can result in fluctuations in heart rate, blood pressure, and vascular tone, leading to cardiovascular instability.

b. Hypotension and hypoperfusion: Severe head trauma can cause a decrease in blood pressure and inadequate blood flow to vital organs, including the heart. This can result in hypotension (low blood pressure) and hypoperfusion (reduced blood flow), which can lead to organ dysfunction and potential cardiovascular complications.

c. Cardiac arrhythmias: Head trauma can trigger abnormal heart rhythms or arrhythmias. The impact on the electrical conduction system of the heart can disrupt the regular heartbeat, leading to bradycardia (slow heart rate), tachycardia (rapid heart rate), or other irregularities. These arrhythmias can affect the heart's ability to pump blood effectively.

d. Myocardial contusion: In some cases, head trauma can cause direct injury to the heart muscle, leading to a condition known as myocardial contusion. This injury can result in myocardial dysfunction, chest pain, and potential complications such as heart failure or arrhythmias.

e. Increased risk of cardiovascular disease: Studies have shown that individuals who have experienced moderate-to-severe head trauma may have an increased risk of developing cardiovascular disease later in life. The mechanisms behind this association are not fully understood but may involve chronic inflammation, altered lipid profiles, and other systemic changes resulting from the initial head trauma.

3. Chronic stress: Stress is a blanket term for many triggers that alert our bodies that something is amiss. Our nervous system is made up of two states: parasympathetic and sympathetic. The parasympathetic nervous system controls all "rest and digest functions." We need optimal blood flow to be in this state. The sympathetic system controls our fight-or-flight response. If you're hiking in the woods shortly after you've eaten a meal and a bear begins chasing you, the bear will get two meals if he catches you: you as one and your undigested food as dessert. Your body was parasympathetic until the bear appeared and started chasing you. Then your body immediately switched into a sympathetic state to keep you alive. It's an excellent acute solution designed to help you survive. Things go off the rails when we're in a chronic sympathetic state.

Your body can't distinguish between a bear running after you in the woods and your stressed-out reaction to a letter from the IRS saying they will audit you. The brain recognizes both situations as threats and prepares the body accordingly. Pain, fatigue, mental stress, and physical danger all feel the same to your brain. When we have too much chronic stress in our lives, we're locked in a long-term sympathetic state which causes our blood pressure to rise. Part of cracking this code is discovering the triggers that put you in a chronic state of stress. Once we know them, we work hard to diminish or eliminate them.

Treatment for vascular issues depends on the root cause of this often hidden code. However, here are some of the modalities I often suggest to my patients:

1. Laser therapy: This is a great modality for improving blood flow, as well as decreasing inflammation. How does it improve blood flow? Decades of phototherapy research have found that wavelengths of light in the red and infrared bands can be beneficial to living tissue. The light triggers the release of nitric oxide from the blood vessels and red blood cells. Nitric oxide is a molecule that dilates blood vessels and improves vascular activity. Laser therapy also triggers a biological cascade of events that leads to an increase in cellular metabolism and a decrease in both pain and inflammation.

2. Exercising the body. Exercise increases blood flow in the body by several mechanisms. A) Muscle contraction: when you exercise, your muscles contract and relax. This action squeezes the blood vessels in the muscles, forcing blood to flow more rapidly to supply oxygen and nutrients to active muscles. B) Dilation of blood vessels: Exercise releases nitric oxide and causes the blood vessels to dilate. This dilation allows more blood to flow through the arteries, and increase overall blood flow.

3. Exercise for your brain: Exercising your body has many benefits for your brain as well. A) Improve cognitive function: Regular exercise can enhance cognitive abilities such as memory, attention, and problem-solving skills. It stimulates the release of chemicals that promote growth of brain cells called brain-derived neurotrophic factors (BDNF, which we can test with the Cyrex LINX

lab test) and the formation of new neuronal connections known as neuroplasticity. B) Reduce cognitive decline: Engaging in physical exercise throughout your life is associated with reduced risk of age-related cognitive decline and neurodegenerative diseases like Alzheimer's and Parkinson's. C) Improved mood and stress reduction: Exercise releases endorphins, which are natural mood lifters. It also reduces the production of stress hormones such as cortisol, helping to alleviate symptoms of anxiety and depression.

4. Reducing stress. As stated above, physical exercise has numerous benefits to the body and brain. Breathing exercises, also known as deep breathing exercises are extremely beneficial to the brain as well as body and gut health. The ratio for deep breathing is 1 to 2: for every second you inhale, exhale for two seconds. A healthy person should be able to breath in for eight seconds and out for 16 seconds. Do this simple test and see how you perform. Eat a healthy diet. I know, I know, you've heard this over and over, but a healthy diet is a must for a healthy mind, body, and spirit. Get adequate sleep. The human body needs six-to-eight hours of quality sleep per night. Adequate sleep helps reduce stress hormones like cortisol.

5. Malabsorption issues. This is best diagnosed through testing. Test for an A/G ratio (optimal is 1.8 or below). Also test for gluten and casein sensitivity using Cyrex #3x and Cyrex #4. Test for leaky gut using Cyrex array #2 and small intestinal bacteria overgrowth (SIBO) using Cyrex #22.

Don't be one of those people who overlook this often misunderstood code. Do you constantly have freezing hands and feet? Does your spouse jump when you put your cold toes on them at night? Do you have problems regulating your body temperature? Pay attention to these signs. You may not think cold hands and feet are a big deal, but remember, all the healing is in the blood. If you have cold hands and cold feet you are not getting adequate blood flow to the extremities. This may lead to not only cold hands and cold feet, but also numbness, tingling, and pins and needles. Lack of blood flow to the feet may eventually lead to poor wound healing and possibly amputation.

Cold hands and cold feet may also mean cold brain as well. Decreased blood flow to the brain has signs and symptoms such as focus, attention, concentration issues (brain fog), subjective cognitive impairment, and even worse, mild cognitive impairment. One thing I know about complex chronic illnesses: Nothing happens in isolation. What does this mean? It means you don't just have cold hands and cold feet, you may have cognitive decline, gastrointestinal issues, and difficulty sleeping at night. As human beings, we are usually much more motivated by pain than something we perceive as an oddity or strange phenomenon like cold hands, cold feet, numbness, and tingling. Still, nearly all patients I treat for complex chronic illnesses have vascular issues. Their primary symptoms may be cold hands and feet, yet they have no idea how their cognitive decline, bloating, and gastric reflux play a role in this complex issue of vascular dysfunction. Remember, your enteric nervous system needs optimal blood flow and oxygen to function optimally.

Are you hungry for more insights?
Visit www.thecodebreakeronline.com for an even
deeper dive into the subjects covered in this chapter.

CHAPTER TEN

CODE #6 AUTOIMMUNE DISORDERS AND THE 30/70 RULE

"Courage is being scared to death, but saddling up anyway."

—JOHN WAYNE

Autoimmunity is when the immune system mistakenly attacks and damages the body's healthy tissues and organs, perceiving them as foreign or harmful. It occurs when the immune system fails to recognize the body's cells and tissues as "self" and instead launches an immune response against them. This response can lead to chronic inflammation, tissue damage, organ dysfunction and antibody production. What is antibody production, and how can it be tested? Antibody production is a crucial immune response carried out by the body to defend against infections and foreign invaders. Cyrex array #5 is the test we use. It is a multiple autoimmune reactivity screen that assesses auto-antibodies predictive for certain diseases.

This autoimmune code is like having termites in your house. You can't see them in the beginning, but they are sneakily causing severe damage to your home's infrastructure. Termites can attack any room in your home, and once they invade it may take up to five years before damage is apparent. Just like termites eating away at your walls, an autoimmune disorder can attack any tissue or organ in your body. Chronic inflammation (Code #1) is one way to trigger these conditions when the immune system becomes dysregulated and confused.

As a child, we watched the animated cartoon show Looney Tunes, and one of the characters was the Tazmanian Devil, sometimes call Taz. He was generally portrayed as a dimwitted wild animal with a notoriously short temper and little patience. Once irritated, he would go into his "twister" mode and destroy everything in his path. Take Taz, make him mad, and hand him an Uzi machine gun. Now you have an idea of what an enraged immune system can do to your body.

Here's another analogy for you. When an army accidentally injures fellow soldiers, mistaking them for the enemy, it's called friendly fire. An autoimmune disorder works in the same way. The immune system overreacts and goes "FIRE, ready, aim" at everything in its path. In trying to protect you, the immune system gets confused and overwhelmed and attacks not only the invader but your own tissues and organs, destroying the good and the bad guys.

TYPES OF AUTOIMMUNITY

1. Genetic Predisposition: Certain genetic factors can increase an individual's susceptibility to developing auto-immune diseases. Specific genes can influence immune system function and regulation, making some individuals more prone to autoimmune reactions.

2. Environmental Factors: Environmental triggers such as infections, toxins, and exposure to certain medications can initiate or exacerbate autoimmune responses in genetically susceptible individuals. These factors can induce immune system dysregulation.

3. Leaky gut and autoimmunity is the third link to autoim-
    mune diseases. A 2020 research paper from the National
    Institute of Health centers around leaky gut syndrome
    and how it stimulates autoimmune pathogenesis. The
    CliffsNotes summary is: the authors conclude that auto-
    immune disorders are facilitated and fueled by heredity,
    environment, and altered gut microbiota. The traditional
    model of autoimmune pathogenesis relating to particular
    genetic constitution and contact with environmental
    triggers has lastly been challenged by the inclusion of
    a third component: damaged gastrointestinal function.
    They go on to say that gliadin (a type of protein found
    in gluten containing grain, primarily wheat, but also in
    barley and rye) can contribute to the loss of stomach
    wall function and prompt the autoimmune reaction in
    genetically prone people. This is extremely important.
    This recent theory suggests that as soon as the autoim-
    mune process is triggered, it is not auto-continuing, but
    can be moderated, or even overturned, by inhibiting the
    constant interplay between the genetic factors and the
    environment. Basically, identify the triggers, remove the
    triggers, and let the body heal. What a different outlook
    compared to the "Standard of Care" and statements like
    "Sorry we don't know what to do," "Learn to live with
    it," or "It's genetics." Even Taz, known for his destructive
    demeanor, could be rendered docile by the power of
    music.

Let's discuss each of these factors in greater detail, starting
with genetics. We all carry unique genetic information, which
we get from our parents. As autoimmunity is a multifaceted

phenomenon, genetics only contribute 30% to the overall picture of its development. Environmental factors including infections, inflammation, diet, and lifestyle all play a crucial role in the development and progression of autoimmune diseases. And, "leaky gut" adds a third layer of complexity to our understanding of autoimmunity, emphasizing the interconnectedness of the gut, the immune system, and the disease process.

The 30/70 rule: 30 % genetics, 70 % environmental toxins and leaky gut. Epigenetics is the study of how your environment can cause changes that affect the way your genes work, and refers to changes of gene expression that don't involve alterations in the DNA itself. Unlike genetic changes, epigenetic changes are reversible and do not change your DNA sequence. However, they can alter the way your body reads the DNA sequence.

I consistently tell my patients, "Genetics loads the gun. Environment and lifestyle pull the trigger." Let's say you have celiac disease, an autoimmune disorder that primarily affects the small intestine. It's triggered by the consumption of gluten, barley, and rye. Symptoms may include abdominal pain, bloating, gas, indigestion, depression, and anxiety. Your celiac gene (the gun) is always loaded; you've had it from conception. However, your environment and food (gluten, barley, rye) pull the trigger and activate the gene. Guess how you solve this problem? Not with drugs, lotions, or potions. It's with your lifestyle choices and a permanent and lifelong gluten-free diet. In this particular case, celiac disease, which carries with it either the HLA-DQ2 gene or the HLA-DQ8 gene, is turned "on" or "off" by the consumption of gluten.

Another part of the autoimmune equation is molecular mimicry, which is a phenomenon in which certain foreign substances, such as gluten, milk, bacteria, plastics, mold and heavy metals can actually resemble the body's cell proteins. This similarity can confuse the immune system, as it may mistakenly attack a foreign antigen and the body's tissues at the same time. Molecular mimicry is thought to contribute to the development of autoimmunity by triggering an immune response against self.

The best way to explain molecular mimicry is to think of a protein made up of various alphabet letters. For an easy example, think of my name, ANDY, as a protein. Just like my name, a protein is made up of individual letters called amino acids. There's a mortgage banker in Tupelo, Mississippi named ANDI. Both sound exactly the same and the spelling is almost identical. So imagine if she and I were in a crowded room and someone yelled, "ANDY or ANDI." Which of us would look at the person yelling "our" name? Both of us. That's an example of molecule mimicry. Our immune system gets confused when foreign invaders have similar amino acid sequences as our own tissues. Research tells us the amino acid sequence only needs five amino acids in its chain to trigger antibodies against our tissues or organs. Over time, this reaction may lead to an autoimmune disorder.

To give you a specific example, alpha-gliadin, which is part of the gluten family, has an amino acid length of 260–330 amino acids. Your thyroid stimulating hormone (TSH), has 211 amino acids. If just five amino acids are linked similarly, your immune system may launch an attack against alpha-gliadin and your thyroid stimulating hormone at the same time which could lead to an autoimmune thyroid issue known as Hashimoto's.

EXAMPLES OF AUTOIMMUNE DISEASES

1. Rheumatoid Arthritis: an autoimmune disease that primarily affects the joints, causing pain, swelling, and stiffness. It can also affect other organs. When it comes to molecular mimicry, lectins are the biggest culprit. Common dietary sources of lectins include legumes (beans, lentils, peanuts), nuts (almonds, cashews, pine nuts, hazelnuts, sunflower seeds, and sesame seeds), and nightshade vegetables such as tomatoes, potatoes, and peppers. Due to molecular mimicry, some studies have suggested that lectins might trigger an immune response in susceptible individuals. Some researchers go as far as calling lectins the "kiss of death" for joints. If you want to learn more about lectins and their connection to auto-immune disease, please read Dr. Aristo Vojdani's book, *Food-Associated Autoimmunities: When Food Breaks Your Immune System.* We can test for this issue using Cyrex array #10. Don't guess: test.

2. Hashimoto's Thyroiditis: an autoimmune disorder that targets the thyroid gland, leading to inflammation and eventual destruction of thyroid tissue. We can test thyroid antibodies using Cyrec Labs array #5.

3. Multiple Sclerosis: an autoimmune disease characterized by inflammation of and damage to the central nervous system. Butyrophilin is a milk protein and is associated with multiple sclerosis. Milk butyrophilin carries molecular similarities to the neurological system and can trick the immune system into attacking the myelin

oligodendrocyte glycoprotein (MOG). We can test for milk butyrophilin with Cyrex Labs array #4.

When you have a full-blown autoimmune disorder, you can never be fully cured of it. However, we can manage it. Lifestyle choices trigger these diseases, and the right decisions can send them into remission. You can manage this code well with the proper tests and strategies. Let me give you an example using celiac disease. If you carry the genetic code for celiac disease, you carry it for life, but you can decide not to eat gluten, remove the trigger, and the gene remains silent.

I help my patients take a proactive approach to autoimmunity using three tests from Cyrex Labs. The first test is array #5, which tells us the tissues that are being tagged with predictive antibodies. The second test is Cyrex array #11, which tells us that environmental triggers may be causing the immune system to go into hyperactive mode. The third test is Cyrex array #12, which identifies the pathogens in the body causing the immune system to be on high alert.

Once you know the triggers of any potential autoimmunity, the goal is to remove or at least minimize them. Ultimately, your lifestyle choices and environmental factors switch these genes on or off.

PATIENT SUCCESS STORIES

My wife, Faye, is my most incredible patient success story because she's the reason I began studying metabolic testing and functional medicine in the first place. I share a bit of her journey with autoimmune disease in my second best-selling book,

Highway to Health: The Road To Overcoming Depression, Anxiety, Insomnia, and Chronic Pain Through the Gut-Brain Connection. The following section is an excerpt from *Highway to Health,* which you can find on Amazon.

****

Imagine spending four years attending chiropractic college, practicing as a chiropractor for five years, and then dedicating six years to studying for a diplomate and fellowship in functional neurology, only to discover I *still* didn't have the answers I needed to heal the person I love most: my wife, Faye. That was an eye-opening realization for a doctor who prided himself on being current with the latest medical research. It was also very motivating. For several years, Faye had struggled with her thyroid. She also had an autoimmune-based skin problem, known as vitiligo. While these issues didn't prevent her from doing the things she wanted to do, I knew there had to be underlying causes that weren't being addressed.

Yet, I didn't just lack answers for Faye's condition. There were patients coming into my clinic for neurological treatment that clearly had autoimmune struggles too. I was helping them improve their neurological issues, but I knew that to achieve true health and vitality, and to optimize their recovery they must be set free from the autoimmune dysfunction that held them back. I had a choice to make: Either bury my head in the sand and continue treating everything like a neurological problem, turning a "blind eye" to the metabolic aspect of health care *or* face the reality that I needed to ask new questions to solve these health problems. Ultimately, my desire to help Faye and my patients sent me back to a place with which I was familiar:

school. I chose to return to the Kharrazian Institute, this time to study functional medicine. I knew someone out there had the answers I sought, and I was determined to find them.

My functional medicine studies led me to ask new questions, discover new philosophies, and finally uncover the hidden key I'd been seeking. I'd studied the brain extensively while earning my diplomate and fellowship in functional neurology through the Carrick Institute, but my true "Eureka" moment came when I learned of the existence of the brain-gut connection. Talk about a light bulb experience! The brain and the gut (essentially, the digestive system) are connected by the vagus nerve (known as "the Wanderer"). It's the longest and most complex of the 12 pairs of cranial nerves. It acts as a superhighway of connectivity between the brain and the gut, and vice versa.

I learned that most chronic neurological disorders actually originate in the gut *first*, then manifest in the brain. Here existed a superhighway of communication, connectedness, and a relationship between the gut and the brain that I'd *known about before, but never really understood.* Here was the answer! My desire to help Faye with her autoimmune condition turned into an epic journey of learning and re-arranging all the health paradigms I'd previously known, and this gut-brain connection was the key I needed to help my patients unlock their full potential for health, healing, and vitality.

Through my studies of functional medicine and the gut-brain connection, I began to learn about "leaky gut," a digestive condition that allows undigested proteins, bacteria, toxins, and gluten to "leak" through the intestinal wall into the sterile bloodstream. I discovered that this seemingly simple condition can lead to an inflammatory cascade and possibly trigger an autoimmune reaction in the brain, gut, and body. My paradigm continued to expand and shift as I realized that Faye's auto-immune conditions were likely being triggered by our *diet* and *environment*. I also learned that gluten, a protein found in wheat, barley, and rye, was one of the most vicious culprits in causing leaky-gut, inflammation as well as autoimmunity because most people genetically cannot digest the modern forms of gluten so common in our food.

During my studies, I was introduced to Enterolab: a lab that tests for the gluten gene as well as the celiac gene and malab-sorption issues. Test results show A) if you carry the gene(s) for gluten intolerance and B) if the gluten gene(s) have been turned on and are currently active, potentially damaging your tissues and organs. I encouraged Faye to take this test, and I decided to take it as well, to be a supportive husband of course. When the results came back, I was shocked. Not only did Faye have the gene for gluten intolerance *and* it was turned on, but *so did I*, only my symptoms hadn't manifested yet. Talk about a slap in the face! I thought I was being a hero by supporting my wife, and it turned out I *too* had a gluten sensitivity disorder.

This was another turning point in my journey both as a doctor and as a person seeking vibrant, long-lasting health. I had a choice to make: Would I ignore the science and the lab results and continue living my life the way I always had? Or would I get ahead of this inflammatory process before it turned into a potential autoimmune condition and "head it off at the pass" by radically changing my diet and lifestyle? Faye and I had to ask ourselves the same question I now ask all of my patients, "How far are we willing to go? What are we willing to do to fix this problem for good, optimize our health, and live life to its fullest?"

We wanted to be well and decided we were willing to do what it took to ensure that would happen. Once I understood the powerful connection between the brain and the gut via the vagus nerve, major changes began to happen. We not only needed to optimize our brain function, but we also needed to heal our guts. This meant making some major lifestyle changes.

For starters, we completely eliminated all gluten from our diet. We also embarked on a 10-week program called the Brain and Body Detox. These two changes kickstarted the healing of our leaky guts and helped decrease the inflammation in our bodies. Faye is a wonderful cook and she immediately got to work learning how to make all of our family's favorite foods using gluten-free flour. Like everyone who undertakes a major lifestyle change, we went through our share of "learning experiences," trials, and tribulations as we adjusted to our new normal. One of my favorite stories from this season involves Faye's first experiments making homemade, gluten-free biscuits. She and I were both surprised when they came out looking (and tasting) like hockey pucks rather than fluffy, flaky Southern-style biscuits. Now we can laugh about the hockey puck biscuits, but like anyone learning something new, we made a lot of mistakes. The difference is that we didn't let it discourage us or make us give up. We learned from those mistakes, fixed them, and kept moving forward—and so can you!

****

For patients who suffer from Hashimotos, most healthcare professionals don't run the appropriate tests. Many test for TSH, T4, and T3, but in my clinic, we test for thyroid antibodies. Through this testing, we can see if your thyroid is undergoing an autoimmune attack. As I mentioned earlier, gluten is one of the biggest culprits of thyroid issues because gluten and thyroid tissue share a few of the same letters in their protein sequences. Fatigue, mental sluggishness, and focus, attention, and concentration problems are one of the earliest signs that gluten is triggering an autoimmune reaction in your body. The cerebellum, the part of your brain responsible for coordinated movements, balance, language, attention, vision, and eye movements, shares a few letters in its amino acid code with gluten, making it a target for an out-of-control immune system that's angrily trying to track down and destroy gluten proteins.

This is why I leave no stone unturned when breaking my patients' unique code of complex chronic illness. I know what it's like to watch someone you love dearly struggle with the heartbreaking realities of poor health and compromised mental acuity because of an autoimmune disorder. Still, there is hope because we can find autoimmune issues years before they become full-blown problems. Your code isn't the same as your neighbor's code or Faye's code. What drives one person's autoimmunity doesn't cause another person's disease.

Unfortunately, autoimmunity is becoming more and more prevalent, and the "standard of care" isn't cutting it anymore because it doesn't look at most of the tests I've shared in this chapter. They're all within the realm of "exceptional care," and the "standard of care" falls sadly short. I have helped people struggling with autoimmunity to reclaim their lives back because they were ready to make the lifestyle changes. They were willing to take total responsibility for their health. If they only want to chase the standard of care, I can't get them the desired results. It isn't enough when we rely on someone else's decisions to fix our health problems. People with complex chronic illnesses suffer because they probably see doctors who only offer the standard Western medicine approach. This doesn't cut it for chronic disease. I see patients recover their vibrance, joy and hope when they step up, take control of their health, and become their own heroes and code-breakers.

STAGES OF AUTOIMMUNITY:

Stage 1: The patient has elevated antibodies against a particular tissue, but no symptoms yet.

Stage 2: The patient has elevated antibodies with symptoms, but not enough tissue destruction to receive a diagnosis.

Stage 3: The patient has elevated antibodies, symptoms, and tissue destruction. It's important to point out that a person can stay in stage one or two for as long as 20 years, going from doctor to doctor seeking answers. Yet all that may have been needed was the predictive antibody test, which is Cyrex array #5.

Below is an autoimmunity case study submitted by one of my Barlow Brain and Body Institute students, Dr. Brian Petrie. It's an excellent example of this important code-breaking work which can help patients regain their quality of life.

****

One of the profound benefits I received from training with Dr. Andy Barlow and from the education at the Barlow Brain and Body Institute was how to work through complicated cases and apply critical thinking skills, an art that appears to be fading in our modern healthcare system.

Laura was a 54-year-old female who originally came to see me because of her chronic joint pain. She stated that her knees were her worst problem. She had gone to orthopedic doctors who performed cortisone injections, which only provided temporary relief. The doctor said she was bone-on-bone and needed knee replacement surgery. Wanting to avoid surgery is what brought Laura to my office. When we first met, it was evident in her case history that her problem was not isolated to her knees. She revealed to me that she was suffering from chronic digestive issues, unexplained weight gain, lack of energy, and brain fog, and she did not feel like herself. She said, "It feels like I'm in someone else's body."

It was clear that she was suffering from an underlying metabolic disorder, which was the likely cause of all her symptoms. As I dug deeper into her history, she revealed that she was employed at a local Home Depot and in the Garden department, where she frequently handled plants and dirt.

I explained to Laura that there was likely a high level of chemical exposure from her employment, particularly when handling the commonly known pesticide Round-up, AKA glyphosate, which is known to destroy the gut and mucosal barriers, often resulting in intestinal permeability. In addition, I explained to her that there tends to be a high level of mold in the dirt, and she likely had frequent exposure. The good news was that she no longer worked there. However, she probably suffered from these long-term effects after seven years of employment.

I told her that these exposures might have caused an excessive toxic chemical load on her body, and that load could have triggered her immune system to become hyperactive and attack her body's tissues, which is a condition known as autoimmunity. In addition to her findings, I noted on physical examination that I was most concerned that she had an autoimmune attack against her thyroid gland and that we needed to do the appropriate lab tests to confirm a working diagnosis.

When I received her results from the labs, it was clear that she had autoimmune antibodies against her thyroid gland, which was consistent with Hashimoto's thyroiditis. This condition was the likely cause of her vast symptoms. I performed additional lab tests to determine the triggers that drove her immune system to become hyperactive. Because of what she revealed in her history, I completed a Cyrex #2 leaky gut panel. This test showed a significant breach in her gut barrier, likely due to the repeated exposure to Round-up. A mold panel also revealed high levels of several multi-cell mold species.

I told her that we needed to eradicate the mold from her body and repair her leaky gut, as these were the primary triggers I found activating her immune system while providing thyroid support if we were ever to change her life and keep her health from spiraling downward.

After three months of a gut repair program, the proper mold protocol, and thyroid support, Laura had a drastic turnaround in her health. She stated that her brain fog had wholly resolved, she lost much of her unwanted weight, her energy levels returned, her digestive function was back to normal, her joint pain resolved, and she no longer needed knee replacement. One of the last things she told me was, "I feel like a new woman."

Dr. Brian Petrie
Raynham, Massachusetts

Are you hungry for more insights?
Visit www.thecodebreakeronline.com for an even
deeper dive into the subjects covered in this chapter.

CHAPTER ELEVEN

CODE #7 TRAUMA

*"It's your life; you don't need permission
to live the life you want."*

—ROY BENNETT

The Oxford Dictionary defines trauma as "a deeply distressing or disturbing experience." In the context of medicine, it's called "physical injury." We will discuss both kinds of trauma and how the brain processes both. Although the brain does not process emotional and physical pain identically, research on neural pathways suggests a substantial overlap exists between the experience of them. With such an overlap, it can be seen that both traumas have a detrimental effect on various areas of the brain, especially the amygdala, hippocampus, and prefrontal cortex.

The amygdala plays a crucial role in processing emotion, particularly the formation and storage of emotional memories. For example, as you walk into a bakery, the smell reminds you of your grandmother's chocolate chip cookies. The amygdala can store happy memories or sad ones. It can also contribute to the regulation of emotional responses including fear, aggression, and rage. It is also involved in assessing the emotional significance of sensory information and can trigger the body's "fight or flight" response when it perceives threat.

The hippocampus is a vital structure in the brain, primarily responsible for several key functions related to memory and spatial navigation. Its functions include:

1. Memory Formation: The hippocampus is crucial for the formation of new declarative or explicit memories. It helps consolidate information from short-term memory to long-term memory.
2. Spatial Navigation: The hippocampus plays a role in spatial memory, allowing individuals to navigate their environment and remember spatial relationships between objects and places.
3. Memory Retrieval: While the hippocampus is important for forming memories, it is also involved in the retrieval of stored memories, helping us recall past experiences and information.
4. Learning: The hippocampus is essential for learning, as it enables the encoding and retention of new information, which is critical for various tasks.

Damage or dysfunction of the hippocampus can lead to memory problems and difficulty with spatial orientation, as seen in conditions like Alzheimer's and amnesia.

The prefrontal lobes, located at the front of the brain, are responsible for a wide range of complex cognitive and executive functions, including:

1. Executive Functioning: The prefrontal cortex is involved in higher-order executive functions such as planning, decision-making, and problem-solving. It helps individuals set goals, make choices, and execute plans.
2. Attention Control: The prefrontal lobes play a role in focusing on and sustaining attention on the task at hand

3. Working Memory: It plays a crucial role in working memory, which is the ability to temporarily hold information in your mind, essential for tasks like mental arithmetic or following instructions. Looking back at the seven stages of Alzheimer's, we can see how the prefrontal lobes control attention as well as working memory, playing a part of stages two, three, and four.

4. Emotional Control and Regulation: These lobes play a role in regulating and controlling our emotions. They help us manage and adapt our emotional responses in various situations. In other words, the prefrontal lobe, when healthy, inhibits the emotion center of the brain: the amygdala.

5. Social Behavior: The prefrontal lobes contribute to our ability to understand and interact with others. They are involved in social cognition, empathy, and interpreting social cues, which are crucial for maintaining relationships.

When an individual experiences prefrontal lobe trauma, neuroinflammation, or neurodegeneration, they may exhibit various signs and symptoms. These can include difficulties with focus, attention, concentration, and memory—such as walking into a room and forgetting their intentions. They may also experience cognitive rigidity, finding it challenging to adapt to new ideas and situations. Additionally, they may have a preference to solitude, feeling the need to withdraw from social interactions. Please understand; these symptoms can vary from person to person.

Like an acute inflammatory response in the body, the brain has God-given, innate strategies for handling the effects of trauma. One such strategy is microglial cells. They are a type of immune cell found in the central nervous system, specifically the brain and spinal cord. They regulate brain development, maintenance of neuronal networks, and injury repair. They're the housekeepers of the brain. In ideal conditions, they're not intended to work all the time. They're only supposed to act when the brain is injured and needs repair.

Due to brain trauma—either head injury or chronic phys-iological stress—the microglial cells can turn from helpful housekeepers to tiny destroyers. When they become overactive or dysfunctional, they can release even more harmful substances that lead to even more chronic inflammation and damage to sur-rounding neurons. This chronic inflammation can disrupt nerve transmission, causing a slowdown in brain activity leading to focus, attention, and concentration issues as well as depression and anxiety.

And there's more: Brain inflammation can disrupt the brain-gut axis by altering the communication between the brain and gut via the vagus nerve. To learn more about this subject, please refer to my second number-one best-selling book. *Highway to Health: The Road To Overcoming Depression, Anxiety, Insomnia, and Chronic Pain Through the Gut-Brain Connection.* Here's a quick overview: Inflammation in the brain can lead to the release of proinflammatory molecules that can negatively affect the integrity and function of the gut lining. This disruption can result in changes in gut permeability, aka leaky gut, leading to imbalances in gut bacteria, small intestinal bacterial overgrowth (SIBO), and alterations in the production of neurotransmitters and hormones involved in the gut-brain axis signaling. The super highway connecting the gut-brain axis is the vagus nerve.

You may be asking how long microglial cells stay activated. It can vary depending on the specific context and underlying cause, as well as the health and lifestyle of the individual. In acute conditions such as injury or infection, they may stay activated for a short period, typically days to weeks, if the individual responds to immediate treatment. If the individual does not respond to immediate treatment and reduce inflammation, chronic neuroinflammation may lead to neurodegenerative changes. Symptoms may include chronic headaches, nausea, brain fog, gastrointestinal issues, bloating, gastric reflux and more. In a chronically inflamed state, the microglial cells can remain activated for months even years.

After an automobile accident or head injury, the primary goal of emergency room staff is to provide life-saving care. If there are no apparent signs of severe injuries such as broken bones, lacerations, dislocations, or hemorrhages, they may discharge you and assure you that everything seems fine—at least at the surface level. However, neuroinflammation maybe occurring, and it's important to know that some injuries may not be immediately evident, but will manifest symptoms over time. I often say to my patients, "Tell me about your first car wreck." They will sometimes give me a funny look and ask, "What does my car accident from 20 years ago have to do with my headaches, anxiety, brain fog ,and chronic pain?" My answer: "Everything."

I know it may be challenging for most to realize that an event which happened years or decades ago can still have a significant impact on their health today. However, the aim of this chapter is to shed light on the profound effects of trauma and how it triggers neuroinflammation, and to emphasize the importance of taking this condition seriously.

FOUR WAYS HEAD TRAUMA CAN IMPACT YOUR LIFE

1. Focus and Attention: Head trauma can disrupt cognitive processes, including focus and attention. The injury can cause difficulties with concentration, reduced attention span, and problems with information processing. This can significantly impact daily activities and cognitive performance.

2. Concentration: Following head trauma, individuals may experience difficulties with concentration. They may struggle to sustain attention on tasks, easily get distracted, or have problems with multitasking. Cognitive impairments and disruptions in neural networks due to the injury can contribute to these concentration difficulties.

3. Chronic Pain: Head trauma, especially if it involves injury to the neck or head structures, can lead to chronic pain. Persistent headaches, migraines, neck pain, and other types of pain, such as fibromyalgia, can occur due to the trauma. The mechanisms underlying post-traumatic pain are complex and involve both peripheral and central sensitization processes.

4. Leaky Gut: The gut-brain connection is bidirectional, and head trauma can disrupt the gut barrier function, leading to increased intestinal permeability, often called "leaky gut." Inflammatory responses triggered by head

trauma can affect the integrity of the gut lining, allowing toxins, bacteria, and other molecules to enter the bloodstream. This can contribute to gastrointestinal symptoms, systemic inflammation, and potential long-term health consequences.

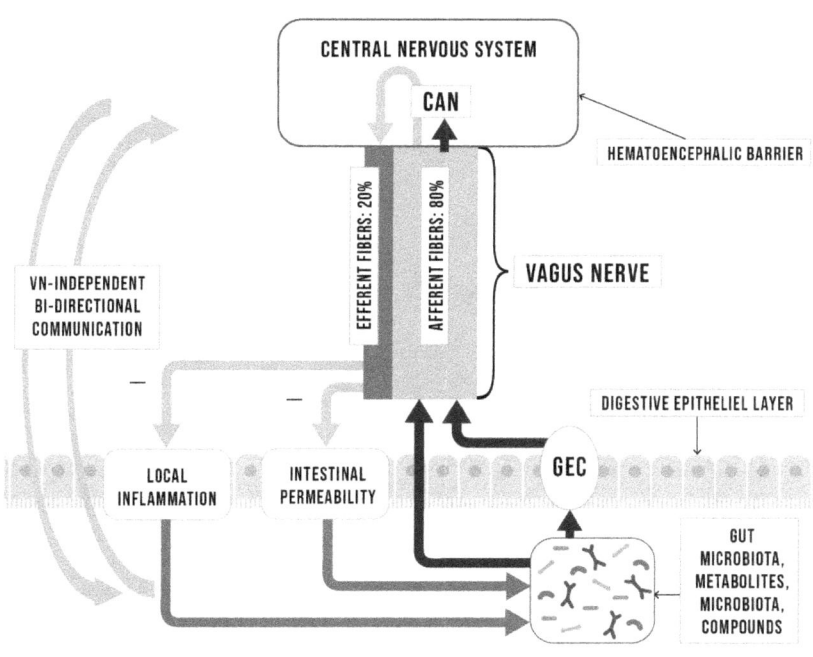

Are you hungry for more insights?
Visit www.thecodebreakeronline.com for an even deeper dive into the subjects covered in this chapter.

PART THREE

UNDERSTANDING YOUR NEXT STEPS

CHAPTER TWELVE

THE SEVEN PRIMARY PATIENTS

"Everything you want is on the other side of fear."

—UNKNOWN

After learning about the seven codes to complex chronic illness, have you noticed any of them in your life? We've talked about the codes individually, but I want to share more about how each code might manifest in your day-to-day activities. When dealing with intricate, complex chronic illnesses, it is important to remember that individuals are not limited to a single code. Instead, there exists a complex combination of codes, each with its own varying degree of severity. Understanding these seven codes and how they manifest in your daily life empowers you to become your own code breaker. By identifying and eliminating these codes, you can begin the process of healing your body, putting together the pieces of the puzzle, and restoring your well-being.

THE INFLAMED PATIENT

If you suspect you have chronic inflammation, signs and symptoms may include joint pain, brain fog, gastrointestinal issues, fibromyalgia, or chronic headaches. The easiest way to confirm your hunch is through a blood test. A standard blood panel should show you most of the markers I mentioned in chapter one. Your hemoglobin A1C should be no higher than 5.3 % on that blood test. If it is, you may have a combination of chronic inflammation as well as pre-diabetes or diabetes. If your c-reactive protein levels, measured in milligrams per liter (mg/l), are above 1.0 mg/L, you're inflamed. If your homocysteine level, measured in micromoles per liter (mcmol/l,) is above 7 mcmol/L, you have inflammation in your body. If your A/G ratio is above 1.8, you're inflamed. An A/G ratio above may also indicate malabsorption as well as liver or kidneys issues. Blood tests help objectify your reality. You can finally say with certainty, "Yes, I am in pain. I am suffering from chronic inflammation, and I have the lab results to prove it." No more "You're faking it" or "It's all in your head."

Remember, you can have inflammation in your brain, body, or gut, and sometimes all three places. Suppose most of the inflammation is affecting the brain. In that case, the individual comes to the office with focus, attention, concentration issues, depression, anxiety, or insomnia. If his or her chronic inflammation is primarily attacking their body, they may have joint and muscle pain, stiffness, neuropathy, fibromyalgia, or other body pain disorders. If it's settled mainly in their gut, they'll have gastric reflux, stomach pain, bloating, distension, diarrhea, or constipation.

One example of an inflamed patient is a woman who came to my clinic because of gut problems. She experienced years of suffering, money wasted on diagnostic testing and imaging, and still, not one doctor had an answer for her chronic gut problem. However, they did tell her, "Go home," "You're fine," "There's nothing wrong with you," and "You're just looking for attention." A family member referred her to me, and when she came to my clinic for an exam, she stated that she also had depression, anxiety, and chronic pain. She had systemic inflammation in her brain, body, and gut, and all of her chronic problems were linked to this code: inflammation. Please don't forget, when it comes to complex chronic health issues, nothing happens in isolation. This patient had multiple health issues in her brain, body, and gut stemming from chronic inflammation.

THE BLOOD SUGAR DYSREGULATED PATIENT

The symptoms of blood sugar dysregulation are among the easiest to identify. If your blood sugar is high, you'll feel sleepy or tired after eating a large, high-carbohydrate meal. Take note if you always reach for a coffee or energy drink in the afternoon. That's another sign. This happens because after you eat, your blood sugar rises. If you're insulin resistant, which means your blood sugar is chronically high, your body wants to remove the excess glucose from your bloodstream. It does this by converting glucose into triglycerides. This conversion of glucose to triglycerides requires an enormous amount of energy. Hence, the after-meal nap.

If your glucose levels are consistently between 100 and 125, you're insulin resistant, also known as pre-diabetic. If your blood sugar is consistently above 126, you're officially diabetic. When you have chronic high blood sugar, it wreaks all kinds of havoc in the brain, body, and gut.

High blood sugar levels can negatively impact brain functions in several ways:

1. Cognitive decline: Research has shown that individuals with diabetes are at higher risk of experiencing cognitive

decline and Alzheimer's disease. High blood sugar levels can lead to neuroinflammation and damage to blood vessels in the brain, impairing cognitive function.

2. Reduced memory and attention span: Some studies have indicated that diabetes can affect memory and attention. High blood sugar levels can interfere with the brain's ability to form and retrieve memories.

3. Mental health issues: People with diabetes are at a higher risk of experiencing mental health issues such as depression and anxiety.

Diabetes and its negative impact on the body:

1. Cardiovascular complications: Diabetes is a major risk factor for cardiovascular diseases such as heart attack, strokes, and peripheral artery disease. High blood sugar levels can damage blood vessels, leading to atherosclerosis (hardening and narrowing of the arteries).

2. Kidney damage: Diabetes is one of the leading causes of kidney disease. This in turn impairs the kidneys' ability to filter waste products for the blood. This can eventually lead to chronic kidney disease or kidney failure.

3. Nerve damage: Diabetes can cause peripheral neuropathy and numbness, as well as tingling and burning in hands and feet. Additionally, diabetes can also affect the autonomic nervous system, leading to problems with digestion, sexual function and regulation of blood flow.

4. Weakened immune system: Diabetes can weaken the immune system, making individuals more susceptible to infections and slow wound healing.

5. Foot problems: Diabetes can lead to poor blood circulation and nerve damage in the feet, increasing the risk of foot ulcers, infections and in severe cases, amputation.

Diabetes and Gut Health:

1. Gastroparesis: a condition characterized by delayed stomach emptying. High blood sugar levels can damage the nerves that control the muscles in the stomach, leading to slow or ineffective movement of food through the GI tract. This can result in symptoms of nausea, vomiting, bloating, and even feeling full after eating a small meal.

2. Intestinal bacterial overgrowth: Diabetes can disrupt the balance of good and bad bacteria in the intestine, leading to an overgrowth of harmful bacteria. This can result in symptoms of bloating, abdominal pain, and diarrhea.

3. Increased GI Tract Infections: Diabetes weakens the immune system, making individuals more susceptible to GI infections caused by bacteria, viruses and parasites.

4. A great segue to the next code: malabsorption. Diabetes impairs nutrient absorption: Poorly controlling diabetes can affect the absorption of nutrients from the intestines, leading to deficiencies in vitamins, minerals, and other essential nutrients. This can further impact overall health and well-being.

THE MALABSORPTION PATIENT

Digestion is all about breaking down food and transferring it into the bloodstream. When this process goes off the rails, vitamin and mineral depletion can cause many issues. However, the most prominent sign is usually gut issues like bloating, GI pain, gastric reflux, and excessive gas. Let me ask you a question: How is your gut functioning? Are you currently on medications due to GI complications? Maybe proton pump inhibitors like omeprazole or antacids like Tums or Rolaids? Are you taking laxatives like MiraLAX? How is your digestion and gut function when it's unassisted, meaning you're off your meds? That's the test of your gastrointestinal tract's ability to break down food into amino acids, glucose, fatty acids, vitamins and minerals. Without these critical substrates we can't produce enough healthy new cells. Consequently, the body can't heal itself and we eventually fall victim to the chronic disease process.

4. THE VASCULAR PATIENT

High blood pressure is like your body trying to drink from a fire hose, and low blood pressure is like having a water hose that doesn't quite reach the flower bed. You get some water on the flowers, but it's not optimal and your flowers die. Chronic pain and inflammation are two of the most common drivers of high blood pressure because they activate the sympathetic nervous system, which causes your heart rate to rise. When this happens for a short period of time your body can compensate and recover. When it's happening day in and day out, year after year,

Houston, we have a problem. Several factors can contribute to the development of chronic vascular problems:

1. high blood pressure
2. high cholesterol
3. smoking
4. sedentary lifestyle
5. poor diet and
6. chronic stress.

THE AUTOIMMUNE PATIENT

Autoimmunity has three parts:

1. Genetics
2. Environmental toxins
3. Breach of the intestinal barrier system, or the blood brain barrier system or both, also known as the "gateway" to autoimmune disorders.

Genetics are 30% of the equation. Environmental toxins and breach of the intestinal barrier system, aka leaky gut, and leaky brain make up the other 70%.

The study of epigenetics has significant implications for understanding human health and disease. It provides the insight into how environmental factors can influence gene expression and how these changes can lead to the development of diseases. Epigenetics can be influenced by various factors including environmental, intestinal permeability, diet, and lifestyle choices. Test and find the triggers; remove the trigger; optimize your life.

This is worth repeating. The three stages of autoimmunity:

1. Silent autoimmunity: The immune system is producing predictive antibodies, but the individual is asymptomatic.
2. Reactive autoimmunity: The immune system is producing predictive antibodies, and now the individual has symptoms, but not enough tissue or organ damage to be diagnosed.
3. Autoimmune disease: The immune system has been producing predictive antibodies for approximately 20 years, and now the individual has enough tissue damage and destruction for a diagnosis to be rendered.

It could take 20 years to move from stage one to stage three. My suggestion: don't guess: test with Cyrex array #5.

THE TOXIC PATIENT

The patient's symptoms could be anywhere in the body, brain, or gut. Again, that's why metabolic testing is essential in breaking this code. Cyrex arrays #11 and #12 show the toxins that are causing adverse reactions, and once we have this information, we can minimize or eliminate exposure to them.

THE TRAUMATIZED PATIENT

The traumatic event could be physical trauma, like a car wreck or sports injury, or mental or emotional trauma, like an abusive relationship, divorce, or the death of a loved one. Whichever the trauma, it can trigger neuroinflammation and cause the immune system's microglial cells to overreact and not turn off. Eventually, homeostasis is disrupted. In most people with trauma-related health problems, the event and the symptoms are spaced far apart—sometimes decades. It's hard for these patients to accept that an event which happened 20 years ago has everything to do with their pain and suffering today. After experiencing a significant traumatic event, it would be advisable to consider reevaluating metabolic tests due to the potential impact of the trauma-induced inflammatory cascade on physiological processes within the body. This is because traumatic events can lead to changes in the body's overall functioning, including metabolic processes. By reevaluating metabolic tests, we can have a better understanding of any alterations in metabolic markers, which can provide valuable insights into an individual's health status following a traumatic event.

Are you hungry for more insights?
Visit www.thecodebreakeronline.com for an even
deeper dive into the subjects covered in this chapter.

CHAPTER THIRTEEN

CRACKING YOUR CODE

"Each person must live their life as a model for others."

—ROSA PARK

Since starting my practice in 2001, I've learned to always keep an open mind. Time and experience have taught me that every patient has a different underlying primary code that needs breaking. Even if their symptoms are the same as another patient, their code is unique and needs to be treated as such. This approach respects the patient's individuality and hears their story with an open mind.

Doctors are usually trained with protocols. You get labeled with a named disease process if you have enough tissue or organ damage, if not you maybe be labeled as "looking for attention," or "it's all in your head." Then you're prescribed an FDA-approved drug to treat that disease process, which doesn't address the underlying root issue. Some patients come to me taking 10-to-15 medications, all of which stifle their symptoms, but none that heal their root issues. It's like treating the tip of the iceberg and ignoring the colossal belly underneath the water.

The standard of care and its protocols, drugs, and surgeries works for some people. It truly does help them. But it doesn't work for everyone. So what should patients do when they fall into the second category? When they have no options? For me, it boils down to two things: 1) What is the purpose of being a doctor? It's to do no harm and serve the patient well. As doctors, we are responsible for reading scientific research and keeping an open mind. Each patient has a unique story and life experiences, so why don't they deserve an individual treatment plan? I believe they do. That's where being a "code breaker" kind of doctor is essential. My job is to recognize any neurologic and metabolic codes that are showing in their lab work and neurologic exam and then find the right treatment plan to help their body heal and reach its most tremendous potential.

2) As a doctor, it's my job to keep my ego in check and always do what is best for the patient. It's important to learn and then apply the latest scientific research. I need to find the root cause, not just treat the symptom. To offer exceptional care that changes lives, I need to break the code and create a plan that brings healing and health.

Just because you've been told you must "live with" your chronic health problems doesn't mean you're out of options. If you've been told by a doctor, "This is all in your head," or "Nothing is wrong with you," you've had the wrong people on your team. Those statements mean, "I don't know enough to explain what's wrong with you." So instead, they are blaming it on you.

If they're a medical doctor, they're a learned person in the field of disease care. But to be diagnosed with a disease, you need a certain amount of tissue damage to receive your proper diagnosis. We want to catch these complex chronic illnesses before they're far enough along to have labels. What do you do when the MRIs and CT scans show nothing? When the lab results are just outside of the "normal" range? You need a doctor who believes you, listens to you, and knows how to deal with these issues and catch things early. If you know something is off, find a doctor like me who will hear you out, take you seriously, and help you crack your code and heal.

One of my patients entered the clinic with all the signs of Parkinson's disease—except he had no tremors, which are absent in approximately 30% of Parkinson's patients. He'd been to numerous doctors, and no one could tell him what was wrong. I did his lab tests, and the results came back so bad that it may have been the worst blood work I've seen in the history of my practice. His blood sugar was elevated and multiple inflammatory markers were positive. He had gluten and casein sensitivity, leaky gut, and leaky brain. He also had predictive antibodies to alpha-synuclein (a major constituent of Lewy bodies and a pathogenic hallmark of Parkinson's disease, dementia with Lewy bodies and multiple systems atrophy. So why was he missed? Because he didn't have the telltale signs of Parkinson's. He didn't have tremors, so they told him he was fine.

The question always comes back to "What do you do when traditional medicine fails?" That's the key. This book is written for people who want to get better and need hope that it's possible. If you know you have a problem but have been to the doctor without any answers, this message is for you. You probably picked up this book because you have a chronic issue that's not going away. To get better results, you need better strategies. This is your sign to go somewhere with a different mindset and training to find out the codes that you have and need to be broken.

In the past chapters, we've gone through the seven major codes linearly, but remember: No one has just one code when suffering with complex chronic illness. Every person has a combination of all seven. In almost all cases, there is an overlap between the codes. This is why you need a doctor who knows how to unlock each code individually and understands how they interact.

"Flying Machines Which Do Not Fly" was an editorial published in the New York Times on October 9, 1903. The article predicted it would take one-to-ten million years for humanity to develop an operating flying machine. It was written in response to Samuel Langley's failed airplane experiment two days prior.

Only nine weeks after the article was written, two brothers on December 17, 1903 in Kitty Hawk, North Carolina changed the world as we now know it. Thank you to Wilbur and Orville Wright for never listening to the nay-sayers and critics, and never bending to conventional wisdom. They paid no attention to what "couldn't" be done, and consequently, they changed the world: forever.

To everyone who bought and read my book, I sincerely thank you. Please become your own code breaker and live your life to the fullest.

Yours in Health,
Dr. Andy Barlow, D.C.

ABOUT THE AUTHOR

Dr. Barlow has been in private practice in Tupelo, MS since June 2001. He is a national and international lecturer and educator in the area of Functional Neurology. Dr. Barlow is the lead U.S. instructor for the Trigenics Institute as well as the American Functional Neurology Institute. Dr. Barlow is a Board-Certified Chiropractic Neurologist and a Fellow of the American College of Functional Neurology. Dr. Andy Barlow is a graduate of Pontotoc High School, Itawamba Community College, and received his doctorate in chiropractic at Life University in Marietta, GA. He served four years in the U.S. Navy, stationed in Great Lakes, IL, Yokosuka, Japan on board the aircraft carrier USS Midway CV-41 as well as aircraft carrier in Coronado, CA on board the USS Constellation CV-64. Dr. Barlow received his honorable discharge from the U.S. Navy June 1986. To contact Dr. Barlow, please call him and his team at the Chiropractic Neurology Center of Tupelo at 662.844.1414 or email Dr. Barlow at askdrbarlow_afni@yahoo.com.

TESTIMONIALS
FOR HEALING

"I have to share my excitement and enthusiasm for the breadth and depth of knowledge I have gained to achieve amazing results with my complex chronic condition patients from the Barlow Brain and Body Institute! You know, pretty much any doctor can claim to teach, but few have the mastery and experience from the trenches.

Dr. Barlow values being an exceptional expert, so much so that he consistently studies and researches to bring the newest advancements to both his patients and those of us studying with him. I can say this with absolute certainty because my husband and I have been consistently training with him for a decade. Doctors and patients, the path to recovery from complex chronic health challenges starts here. Dive into this book. There is hope and a way forward."

—DR. SHELLY DRANKO, DC

"Having practiced for 45 years I have had the opportunity to train under numerous great instructors, and I can honestly say now that Dr. Andy Barlow with the Barlow Brain and Body Institute is head and shoulders above them all. I have been following his guidance since 2008 and all I can say is WOW, what a fun ride it has been. The sheer confidence he gives me in how to handle almost every patient that walks through my door is awesome.

He showed me how to run a total cash practice with no insurance so I can provide the best patient care, and how to talk to patients and be able to explain their exam and the importance of taking action before their chronic condition totally destroys their quality of life. He taught me how to fully evaluate the whole patient sitting in front of me and not just their 'Blinky Light' complaint as he calls it. What I really love is that Dr. Andy is constantly evolving; he is never satisfied and is always looking for better ways. And best of all I think of Andy as a great friend."

—DR. JACK GORLESKY, DC

"I had been experiencing leg and chronic knee pain for some years. My doctor referred me to an orthopedic doctor in Birmingham. He took X-rays and told me that knee surgery was my only option for relief. Because I had recently experienced surgery, I was not mentally nor physically ready for more.

Again, consulting with my primary doctor, he referred me to another doctor, a neurologist in Tuscaloosa. I began treatment with him in which he gave me a series of tests for nerve damage in my legs. The results came back very dismal. He said that the veins in my legs were so damaged that he was amazed I could still walk without assistance. This was six months ago. He prescribed Gabapentin and wanted to see me back in six months.

In the meantime, a church member told me how her son had received significant relief from some of the same problems of chronic knee pain and neuropathy from a doctor in Tupelo. This doctor was Dr. Andy Barlow. I made an appointment and went to see him. After he examined me and took some test, he said he was convinced that he could help me without surgery. With the information he presented, showing me my X-rays, and hearing the testimonials of others in the clinic who witnessed how he had helped them, I knew his plan was well worth giving a try. For the next six months, I received treatment from Dr. Andy Barlow.

After six months, it was time for me to go back to see my neurologist in Tuscaloosa. Again, he took the same test to see how much nerve damage had progressed in my legs.

I was still having neurotrophy in my feet and I was convinced that they would be far worse than when he had tested them six months ago. When the doctor entered my exam room with the report, he had sort of a puzzled look and somewhat of a smile. Whichever it was, I immediately looked away, dreading the worst impending news.

The doctor took a seat near me and said, 'Mrs. Sparks, I have some amazing news for you.' He said, 'Mrs. Sparks your test results on your legs show so much improvement from the last test six months ago, that all I can say, it is just short of a miracle.' He continued to say, 'Ninety nine percent of the patients we see with test results like yours would be in a wheelchair by now and yet you are walking and standing, etc. I just don't know how to explain it.' But he said my legs were near normal levels. I could still have neuropathy in my feet, but to have the use of my legs was invaluable.

At this point, the doctor and I were both at the point of tears. My husband told the doctor, 'Well she danced almost half the night away at church giving praises to God, it's no wonder.' I thank God for leading me to Dr. Any Barlow, who has definitely helped me maintain a quality of life that seemingly otherwise I would not have had. I am thankful that Dr. Barlow, through his own personal journey, has gone beyond just accepting the normal trends of medical treatment of 'the pill' and 'the knife' to discover other ways of treatment for his patients that are not so invasive. The treatment that Dr. Barlow has given me has truly helped me.

If this testimonial might encourage or help one person to escape the use of a wheelchair or would ease the painful nights to just being able to get a good night's sleep, than I would encourage you to please schedule an appointment to see Dr. Andy Barlow. He will be honest with you and let you know if he thinks he can help you. For any chronic pain issues, or if you're just not feeling well at all, it will be well worth your time and energy to have a consultation visit with Dr. Barlow at the Chiropractic Physicians Center of Tupelo. My doctor summed it up, 'Your progress is short of a miracle.'"

—MARY SPARKS

"As a retired health care professional, to say the least I was very skeptical of such an approach to health care. With my family's encouragement, and after researching Dr. Barlow, I scheduled an evaluation. During this evaluation my wife and I were impressed with him. We realized how significantly my symptoms had progressed. He made one statement that resonated with me: 'This is not your typical medical care, where you are given a pill to feel better but rather, we are going to figure out what is causing your symptoms and help optimize your recovery.' I felt at this point that here was someone who will leave no stone unturned to determine the cause and resolve my problem.

I have read both his books, and from a scientific point of view the information presented is correct, but also the books were so well written, conveying the information to anyone in an easily understandable way. I further understood that this course of treatment would be a collaborative effort between Andy and me. I would have to learn, adapt to a new way of eating and change my dietary habits for the better as well as for life.

I have been a patient for just under two months and have already seen an improvement in my Symptoms; I fully believe Dr. Barlow will do as he said and help me correct the many issues that have led to my failing health. He has provided me with the information and tools to make the changes required for me to heal and recover. With this help, I hold great hope and aspirations to again enjoy an active life and once again enjoy life to its fullest."

—R.D. ALDRIDGE

"In 2018, I was diagnosed with dystonia, which is involuntary movement of the muscles. My dystonia affects the eye, facial, and neck muscles. I have been prescribed many medicines which have had a negative effect on my memory. I have also had two surgeries: one to implant a brain stimulator. Neither of these helped my situation very much at all.

I had seen Dr. Barlow's ads on TV and thought they were just for muscle and skeletal problems. My husband talked me into going. My first visit was very interesting; Dr. Barlow felt he could help with my disorder. He put me on a detox for 15 weeks and supplied supplements and a guideline to follow. After the first couple of weeks, I started feeling different, and after 10 weeks I was feeling like the old me. I have learned calming exercises that help me when I get stressed that usually bring on the spasms and breathing techniques that also help tremendously.

Looking at the plan, I thought to myself, 'How in the world is this going to help me?' but I can honestly say that my journey has been a major success. I still have issues now and then, mostly brought on by stress or fatigue, but I can also now know how to handle them and change the situation.

I highly recommend Dr. Barlow for your health care needs. I think he is honest enough to tell you upfront whether it's worth it or a waste of time."

—LISA J. FONDREN

"In my career as a healthcare professional, constant learning is pivotal to offering the best care to my patients. However, among the myriad of educators, only a select few can revolutionize a doctor's patient care approach. Andy Barlow is one such exceptional instructor, imparting invaluable lessons at the Barlow Brain and Body Institute.

I had the privilege of meeting Dr. Andy Barlow approximately eight years ago when I undertook his functional neurology certification. Since that pivotal encounter, he has played a crucial role in shaping our doctors into what I term the 'second generation of chiropractic.'

This transformative training has not only elevated our doctors' perspectives and treatment approaches, but has also correlated with a surge in the quality of services and revenue of our practices. Collectively, under the tutelage of one of the chiropractic profession's most esteemed educators, our company has experienced remarkable growth in every dimension."

—DR. TONY DERAMUS

"I had been to the ER twice with my colon being infected in one year. The test showed infection but the cause was unknown. I went to a GI specialist and had a colonoscopy, and was told I had the healthiest colon he had ever seen. Meanwhile I was suffering from debilitating migraines and loss of memory as well as severe depression, and I NEVER felt good. After running into Dr. Barlow at a convention, I called him and asked if he thought he could help me. We scheduled an appointment and I had a thorough examination. At this point my brain was so foggy that I could not drive or remember the name of the hotel that I stayed in. I was scared that something bad was happening and feared that I had dementia. I started the program of care and followed his recommendations; now my brain function is better than it has been in years. I am able to work at a full load again; I no longer suffer from depression and have way fewer migraines. Dr. Barlow truly cares and continues to offer advice on ways to improve my health. I have no doubt that each year I will get better and better. I am amazed at how well I am feeling after years of feeling bad almost every day. God answers prayers! Thank you Dr Barlow."

—DR. SPENCER

"Dr. Barlow and his program, the Barlow Brain and Body Institute, have been instrumental in the success of my practice and the results my patients get. The knowledge I received from attending his training seminars has allowed me to understand better how to communicate with patients and be better at recommending treatments. Dr Barlow has a wealth of knowledge in treating patients and making your practice as successful as possible."

—DR. CLINT FREEMAN

"I'm proud to call Dr. Andy Barlow one of my chief mentors in healthcare. His neuro reconnect techniques revolutionized my clinic's ability to help chronic neurological and musculoskeletal conditions—usually in just a few treatments. Thanks to him, we have hundreds of happy patients who have avoided major orthopedic surgery.

Now, Dr. Barlow is redefining evidence-based care around chronic neurodegenerative conditions like dementia and Parkinson's disease. Using his techniques, our clinic has successfully restored the short-term memory of our first dementia patient, who is 90 years old! Her family is amazed that her memory is improving after being told by her traditional medical providers that she would only continue to worsen. Thank you, Dr. Barlow, for improving the lives of sufferers whom traditional medicine has virtually abandoned."

—ERIC N. CODNER, DC EMT

"Dr. Andy Barlow is a doctor unlike any other. His consistent pursuit of truth and knowledge in healthcare has allowed him to help patients with the most debilitating diseases. Daily, he delivers hope and healing to patients who have repeatedly heard that nothing can be done for them. As a humble and God-fearing man, he truly cares and puts his patients first. I owe much of my clinical success and patient results to Dr. Andy. He is my mentor and friend. Above all, he is a wonderful family man and a light for everyone around him."

—DR. MATTHEW CHRISTENSON

"Dr. Barlow has undoubtedly changed my life. I took him at his word in 2019 and have zero regrets. His groundbreaking work has helped me in so many ways. It has helped me provide more holistic and compassionate care to my patients. His commitment to excellence is unmatched. His passion for helping doctors and patients transform their lives is evident in all he does. Thank you, Dr. Barlow, for dedicating yourself to the well-being of others!"

—DR. JEREMIAH SCHREIBER, Flagship Healthcare, Erie, PA; Gold Coast Regenerative Medicine, Costa Rica

"Before I encountered the work of Dr. Andy Barlow at the Brain and Body Institute, my approach to treating neuropathy was largely reactive, and admittedly less holistic. Dr. Barlow's comprehensive framework for understanding the interconnectedness of neural pathways and overall body health illuminated the root causes of neuropathic pain. His institute's emphasis on the brain-body connection, emphasizing the symptoms and underlying neural dysfunction, allowed me to shift my treatment strategies. By integrating his methodologies, which blend neurology with tailored physical rehabilitation, my patients began to experience more than just symptomatic relief: they began to see a change in their daily functional abilities.

The transformation in my practice became evident as patient outcomes improved significantly. With new diagnostic tools and therapeutic approaches from Dr. Barlow's protocols, I could offer individualized treatment plans addressing specific neural dysfunctions. Patients who had resigned themselves to a life dominated by the limitations of neuropathy started to regain control. Simple joys like walking without pain, improved sleep, and the ability to engage in hobbies became attainable goals. The holistic improvement in their quality of life was physical and emotional, as they found new hope for continued betterment.

The most profound change was the shift in the patient-doctor relationship. Dr. Barlow's teachings taught me the importance of patient education and empowerment. Compliance and optimism soared by involving patients in their treatment plans, explaining the 'why' behind their symptoms, and the 'how' of our interventions. Success stories multiplied, with patients often returning to share how they could now partake in previously impossible activities. Their renewed enthusiasm was a testament to the efficacy of the Brain and Body Institute's approach, and it redefined my practice, turning patient care into a partnership for health and wellness."

—DR. GARRETT GALLENTINE

"Dr. Barlow is genuinely one of a kind. Attending a seminar at his office was pivotal in my professional journey. From the first interaction, I was astounded by his profound understanding of the human body and his remarkable ability to unravel complex cases. His teachings are not just theories: they are practical tools that have revolutionized my approach in my practice. Utilizing his methods, I've managed to turn around challenging cases more effectively, significantly boosting my confidence in approaching patients who have lost hope.

Beyond his expertise, what truly sets Dr. Barlow apart is his dedication. Finding someone so passionately committed to their craft is a rare privilege, especially when their work directly contributes to making the world a better place. His dedication isn't just limited to his professional accomplishments: it extends into his role as a mentor and friend. Learning from Dr. Barlow, I've gained invaluable knowledge and a mentor who genuinely cares about the growth and success of everyone he talks to.

Dr. Barlow's influence on my career has been monumental. His unique blend of expertise, empathy, and dedication makes him an exceptional professional and mentor. I am deeply honored to have had the opportunity to learn from him and to apply his teachings in my practice. His impact extends far beyond his seminars; it resonates in the lives of those he teaches and, subsequently, in the lives of the patients we care for. Dr. Barlow is more than a mentor: he is an inspiration, and his contribution to the healthcare profession is immeasurable."

—DR. JUSTIN WUBBEN

"I had been having issues with my balance for a while, but it began to get **worse** just before beginning treatments with Doctor Barlow. Just before beginning treatments with Doctor Barlow, I had several bad falls. One of these falls was head over heels down a staircase. A couple of the falls resulted in black eyes because I fell face first. Thankfully, I was not severely injured in **any** of these falls, but I was walking with a cane. I had gotten to the point that I couldn't write, type, or text, which impacted my job. I was not able to drive a car. After about a month of treatment with Doctor Barlow, I was able to walk without a cane and text, type, and write. I began driving again a couple of months later. I fully recommend Doctor Barlow's treatment plan."

—KAREN MAXCY

"The decision to see Dr Barlow at his Clinic for memory issues after attending one of his seminars has been life-changing. after seeing traditional medicine fair with several family members, I wanted to be as healthy as possible with a goal to be able to take care of myself throughout the rest of my life.

The test that Dr Barlow used identified gluten sensitivities and food allergies. After making changes in my diet from his recommendations, my mental and physical health have improved. I just wish I had known this early in my life.

Knowledge is powerful. Enhancing your life by eating food without harmful chemical additives has been a great motivator for me. The fact that he and his staff operate using Biblical principles gives me comfort. The treatment at joss Clinic is so helpful at healing your body and mind. I encourage everybody to get Dr Barlow's books and follow his easy suggestions to improve your quality of life. If you can find a way to get a personalized treatment plan at his clinic, you will be blessed."

—PEGGY BURNS

"When I first came to Dr. Barlow's clinic in May 2021, I was using a walker to get around and in extreme pain in the low back, right hip, and right leg. I had been to several neurologists, had shots in the back, and a nerve block. None of it helped the problem so they sent me to pain management. They just wanted to give me more prescriptions. I didn't want anymore drugs. I had heard other people talk about Dr. Barlow's clinic so I decided to give him a try. Within 1 month of coming to Dr. Barlow's clinic I had no pain in my hip or leg and started walking with a cane instead of a walker. I still have some low back pain but that has improved a lot. He did bloodwork and test that no other doctor had ever thought of doing. I did their detox program and supplements. Dr. Barlow has helped tremendously. I am now walking without a cane, standing up straighter, and have more energy! I want to thank Dr. Barlow and all staff for helping me. I would highly recommend Dr. Barlow to anyone that traditional medicine has failed."

—JIM

"The reason I first came to Dr. Barlow was because / was having extreme numbness/tingling in my feet. I was waking up 3 times or more a night to put my feet in hot water to get relief. I had gone to numerous specialists, and no one could tell me what was wrong. I went through nerve conduction studies where the results showed I did not have neuropathy. I couldn't ride in a vehicle hardly any distance at all without major stiffness/pain. Also, I have suffered with lots of gastric problems, and never understood why. No one could tell me. I prayed and prayed about what to do and was led to The Chiropractic Physicians Center. When I got to Dr. Barlow, he did an extensive exam and x-rays that showed I had leaky gut which was causing my severe abdominal pain, among other things. I started his detox program and within 3 days of the detox my gastric problems completely ended. I lost 18 lbs. during the detox. Also recently, I rode from Booneville to Orange Beach and never got stiff or had pain. It was a miracle. What impressed me the most with Dr. Barlow was on the 1st visit he told me he wasn't going to treat the problem; he was here to find the cause of the problem and treat that. I am now sleeping more soundly, not stiff, and my energy levels are unreal! I feel like a whole new person. Anytime

I have had additional problems he acknowledges it immediately. I can't sing his praise enough! I highly recommend Dr. Barlow to everyone. The doctors and staff are wonderful! Dr. Barlow has completely changed my life."

—DIANE R.

"For years, I meandered through the medical system, hearing the same refrain: my balance issues and chronic fatigue were 'normal' and something I just had to accept. But when I met Dr. Andy Barlow, everything changed. From our initial examination, I could sense his approach was different. Instead of dismissing my concerns, he delved deep, unveiling a decades-long issue with my cerebellum that I was completely unaware of. He explained how my gut issues were intricately linked to cerebellum autoimmune problems, a connection no other doctor had ever mentioned to me.

The revelation was profound, but what set Dr. Barlow apart was his ability to communicate complex medical issues in terms a patient could understand. He believes that each person has a unique 'code' that unlocks their healing needs. And for me, he did just that. With his guidance, I began to see improvements that I had only dreamed of.

Thanks to Dr. Barlow, I no longer accept the status quo. He has equipped me with the knowledge and tools to take charge of my health, proving that even the most enduring medical mysteries can be solved with the right person by your side. To anyone seeking answers, I wholeheartedly recommend Dr. Barlow. He is more than just a doctor; he is a healer who can truly unlock the code to your well-being."

—RANDALL CHESNUTT

"Dr. Barlow's book, *Code Breaker*, is the embodiment of brilliance in our profession, a true visionary masterpiece with the potential to revolutionize healthcare as we know it. His innate ability to unravel the intricate code of health and disease and produce innovative solutions is a testament to his genius. In a world where chronic health conditions erode our quality of life and we accept the standard of care to be only symptom relief, Dr. Barlow provides the path to identifying the cause and tools to navigate treatment. His revolutionary approach to health and wellness not only provides life changing results but inspires hope where traditional expectations of healthcare have failed. This third installment in his groundbreaking series once again proves his unparalleled talent to redefine health and our standards of healthcare and inspire the potential to improve lives. The mentorship provided by Dr. Barlow has been instrumental in enhancing my clinical skills and through his guidance, I have been able to bring about significant improvements in my patients' lives and provide hope. The dedication and wisdom of Dr. Barlow is proved through each page of this book making it a must-read for patients and doctors seeking to make a meaningful impact in the world of health and quality of life."

—DR. MARIANNE ABATE, DC, CACCP

"No matter your current health condition, The Barlow Brain and body institute offers a proven framework for improving Chronic health conditions- Andy Barlow, one of the world's leading experts in Neurology and Functional medicine, has revolutionized natural health care.

If you have been suffering with Chronic health conditions such as Chronic pain, thyroid disease Alzheimer, or been told that nothing can be done. You must seek out the Doctor who has been a leader in natural health for over 20 years.

Having trouble changing your health, the problem isn't you. The problem is our healthcare system. Old antiquated treatments and surgeries that don't fix the real cause of your problem. Too many doctors are chasing the blinking light and not addressing the real cause.

Dr Barlow is known for his ability to turn complex conditions into simple solutions that can be easily applied to drastically improve the life of his patients. He draws on the most proven ideas from Neurology and functional medicine to create easy-to-understand treatments for patients that have been forgotten by the medical community. Along the way, Dr Barlow has taught hundreds/ Thousands of doctors around the world how to serve their communities to the highest level. Readers will be inspired and engaged with true stories from people who have suffered far too long. Dr. Barlow has enhanced my life and given me the tools to change the lives of my patients."

—CHRIS STEINER

"My name is Bryce Meredith and in this brief testimonial I will be detailing my journey to recovery from a concussion. For background, I am a 22 year old male and I play division 1 soccer at the University of Memphis. I have never had any diagnosed concussions before, so dealing with one was quite new to me. On June 3rd, 2023, I was playing in a summer league soccer game. A ball was put into the air, and as I jumped to head it away, I was hit with an elbow from the side and I fell backwards and the back of my head hit the ground from about 7 feet up. I was knocked unconscious for around 10-15 seconds, and when I came to I was very disoriented. After a few minutes, I felt decent enough that I decided to go back on the field. Looking back, that was the biggest mistake I made in this whole process. After playing for 5 minutes, I knew something was wrong. I took myself out of the game and rested for the rest of the night. After a few days of taking it easy, I felt somewhat back to normal. The only significant symptom I had was some moderate headaches. After a week and a half, I had been responding pretty well to exercise so I decided I was ready to start playing games again. Another mistake. I ended up playing 2 games while in this state, and it wasn't until after the second game that my symptoms started getting progressively worse. After 2 weeks of symptoms getting worse, I decided to take some time to rest completely. I began seeing a concussion specialist and a chiropractor to treat the concussion and make sure none of my headaches were due to my neck being out of line.

Fast forward to the middle of August, I had been doing plenty of ocular and vestibular exercises along with some chiropractic visits. I had still not gone a day without having moderate headaches. I had never had headaches before the concussion, so I knew things still weren't back to normal. I was starting to get hopeless after 2 months of no progress, and that's when I discovered Dr. Barlow. On my first visit, he conducted an eye exam, balance testing, and a brain map. The results of the testing showed I was pretty far from normal brain function. He prescribed neurofeedback, red laser therapy, and electric stimulation for my legs and feet. He also advised getting a Cyrex blood test, which showed evidence that I had developed leaky gut and had become reactionary to many foods that I had not been reactionary to in the past. Within 4 weeks, my headaches had completely disappeared. At this point, I had been doing the therapies for 4 weeks, and had taken the reactionary foods out of my diet for about 2 and a half weeks. The combination of these things lead to the disappearance of all of my symptoms. After 3 months, I was finally able to get back to playing soccer and functioning normally again. It's now December, and I am happy to report my repeated brain map showed that my brain has almost made a full recovery."

—BRYCE MEREDITH

"I want to express the profound impact that Dr. Andy Barlow and The Barlow Brain and Body Institute have had on my life, both personally and professionally. My journey with Dr. Andy began in 2019 when I first met him at his clinic. Since then, he has been a guiding light in my professional development and understanding of the Regenerative Medicine market.

Professionally, Dr. Barlow has been instrumental in helping me navigate the complexities of the field. He has shown me how to assist other clinicians in integrating their clinics to provide the same hope and healing that he offers to his patients. Dr. Andy's three-pronged approach to healing, encompassing metabolic, neurologic, and regenerative care, serves as a cornerstone of The Brain and Body Institute. His wealth of knowledge isn't just confined to his clinic; he generously shares it with clinicians across the country. What's more, he has the remarkable ability to convey complex concepts in a way that resonates with patients, making them feel that Dr. Barlow is fully committed to their well-being.

On a personal note, Dr. Andy has been a constant source of encouragement in my professional endeavors. When I decided to venture into starting my own business, Dr. Barlow stood by me as my biggest supporter. His keen business acumen has been invaluable, not just to me but also to his colleagues. Dr. Barlow's genuine care for everyone who crosses his path, whether a patient, a fellow physician, or a business associate, is something I've rarely encountered. His kindness and respect leave a lasting impression. I wish Dr. Andy Barlow continued success in all aspects of his life, both personally and professionally. May he continue to be a beacon of hope and healing and may his journey be blessed abundantly."

—CONNIE ESCH

"I had been dealing with numbness in my feet and toe's, along with leg pain for some time, I attempted to address these issues with my primary physician during a wellness exam. There was not much conversation about my concerns, this is something you have to learn to deal with. I was not impressed with this solution, but where do you go for help?

After several month of waiting for things to improve, I decided to contact a foot specialist. X-ray's where taken and I was given some shots between by toes for the pain. The shot given to me gave some relief of my foot pain for a short period. On return to the same doctor for a follow up exam, I was asked how the shots worked. I let him know they helped for a week or so before becoming less effective. Additional shots were offered, to which I declined.

I met with Dr. Barlow a few months later. Once he completed his exam, he said he felt that he could help me to get to the root cause of my issues. His treatment plan required me to make some drastic life changes.

Two months into a nine-month treatment plan, I feel great. My condition has improved drastically. I look forward to the results on completion of the planned therapy. I thank him for showing me how to heal myself to live my best life."

—LARRY WHITE

DR. BARLOW'S RECOMMENDED RESOURCES:

If you would like to hire Dr. Barlow as a key note speaker for your conference, social organization or church please contact a info@BarlowBrianAndBody.com

If you would like to bulk order Dr. Barlow's books for your social group or church please contact info@BarlowBrianAndBody.com

If you would like to set an appointment with Dr. Barlow's clinic please call 662-844-1414

Barlow Brain and Body Institute please go to our website at https://BarlowBrainAndBody.com

Ergo-Flex Technologies- Back on Trac, Knee on Trac, Total Brain and body O2

Linda Anderson 936-201-6923

Shockwave Chuck 561-707-0530

Hakomed Marshall 828-231-7406

Platelet Therapy Connie 508-450-2160

Doctors interested in functional neurology
https://courses.functionalneurologyseminars.com/

Niche-Kings Niche-Kings.com Lindsay
701-941-0008

"I have learned silence from the talkative; tolerance from the intolerant, and kindness from the unkind. I should not be ungrateful to those teachers."

—Kahlil Gibran

PRAYER:

Dear God, help me see that all of my life is a learning opportunity. Please help me to be thankful for both my good and my bad experiences. Remind me that it is through forgiveness that I can become grateful for all the people I have encountered. Today, I will frame all of the past as a learning opportunity. Today, I will remember that I am a student and will remain teachable. Amen.

In memory of Dr. Al Comey, DC, DACNB